MAY 2 3 2016

D0389676

ADVENTURES
OF A FEMALE
MEDICAL DETECTIVE

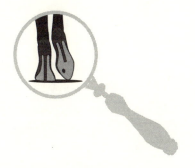

ADVENTURES OF A FEMALE MEDICAL DETECTIVE

IN PURSUIT OF SMALLPOX AND AIDS

Mary Guinan, PhD, MD

with Anne D. Mather

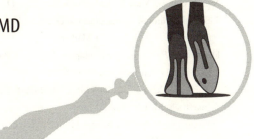

JOHNS HOPKINS UNIVERSITY PRESS
Baltimore

Johns Hopkins University Press
2715 North Charles Street
Baltimore, Maryland 21218-4363
www.press.jhu.edu

Library of Congress Cataloging-in-Publication Data

Names: Guinan, Mary E., author. | Mather, Anne D., author.
Title: Adventures of a female medical detective : in pursuit of smallpox and AIDS / Mary Guinan with Anne D. Mather.
Description: Baltimore : Johns Hopkins University Press, 2016. | Includes bibliographical references and index.
Identifiers: LCCN 2015034008 | ISBN 9781421419992 (hardback) | ISBN 1421419998 (hardback) | ISBN 9781421420004 (electronic)
Subjects: LCSH: Guinan, Mary—Health. | Women physicians—United States—Biography. | Women in medicine—Biography. | Epidemiology—Case studies. | BISAC: MEDICAL / Public Health. | MEDICAL / Infectious Diseases. | BIOGRAPHY & AUTOBIOGRAPHY / Personal Memoirs.
Classification: LCC R692.G85 2016 | DDC 610.82—dc23 LC record available at http://lccn.loc.gov/2015034008

A catalog record for this book is available from the British Library.

Special discounts are available for bulk purchases of this book. For more information, please contact Special Sales at 410-516-6936 or specialsales@press.jhu.edu.

Johns Hopkins University Press uses environmentally friendly book materials, including recycled text paper that is composed of at least 30 percent post-consumer waste, whenever possible.

TO JOAN, BRENDAN, AND CHRISTOPHER

CONTENTS

ACKNOWLEDGMENTS

TO LIBRARIANS Xan Goodman (Health and Science Librarian, University of Nevada, Las Vegas); Terry Henner (Head of Outreach Services, Savitt Medical Library, University of Nevada School of Medicine), who enthusiastically answered every one of my multiple requests for help in finding references and out-of-print books; and Mary Hilpertshauser (Historic Collections Manager, David J. Sencer CDC Museum), who tracked down photos and historical information that were invaluable and is now preserving the history of CDC's contribution to smallpox eradication.

To all my former CDC colleagues who helped me during the writing of this book, especially Harold Jaffe and James Curran, with whom I first worked in the sexually transmitted diseases unit and then transitioned to investigate the emerging AIDS epidemic; Claire Broome, a valued friend and collaborator on the *Listeria* dilemma; Mary Serdula, who shared the assignment in Pakistan and provided photos; Eugene McCray, who led the nationwide "needle-stick" study and helped me find all the relevant papers; Vince Radke, for keeping "smallpoxers" connected; Walter Orenstein, with whom I was assigned to India and shared the joy of discovery of our careers as medical detectives; Helene Gayle, who gave me sage advice I badly needed at various times in my life and encouraged me to write; Verla Neslund, my CDC lawyer, who ably helped me with many tricky legal issues; Wanda Jones, who helped with my testimony on the *Listeria* case; and of course Bill Foege, whose leadership and vision continue to inspire me even after forty years. To my coauthor Anne D. Mather, who was the managing editor of CDC's weekly newsletter, the *MMWR*, when I first met her in 1974, and who edited its article that reported the first cases of AIDS in 1981. Without her persistent encouragement, historical knowledge, good humor, and creative editing, this book would not have been written.

To Gary Wormser, my medical school classmate, with whom I worked when investigating the early AIDS cases in New York and who had the courage to testify in support of John Doe's employment despite the risk to his career. To the anonymous reviewers who convinced Johns Hopkins University Press to publish the book. To the fantastic efforts of JHUP staff: Kelly Squazzo, first acquisition editor; followed by Robin Coleman, who enthusiastically promoted the book and went to extraordinary measures to shepherd it through the system; Isla Hamilton-Short, who was consistently there, especially during the editor transition, to troubleshoot innumerable issues while remaining calm and pleasant; editors Juliana McCarthy and Ashleigh McKown; and our publicist, Kathryn Marguy.

A special acknowledgment to the late Randy Shilts, one of my heroes, who in 1981, during the early epidemic, dedicated his column in the *San Francisco Chronicle* to AIDS, when most other journalists and newspapers avoided AIDS coverage; who wrote the definitive history of the emerging epidemic in *And the Band Played On*, one of the most important books of the twentieth century; and who supported the closing of gay bathhouses in San Francisco, despite vilification by the gay community, because he knew it was the right thing to do to reduce the spread of AIDS.

And finally to my family, especially my niece, Kate Guinan, whose wonderful art enlivens the back cover and interior of the book; my sister Joan Lunney, who when she read my first story told me to "get an editor"; and to my life partner Christopher Horton, who never failed to encourage me.

ADVENTURES
OF A FEMALE
MEDICAL DETECTIVE

Introduction

MANY people have told me that they wished they had known about medical detectives when they were deciding on a career. Until recently, few young people were exposed to medical detective stories or to undergraduate experiences that might have led them to a career as a medical detective, that is, a career in public health.

Epidemiology is the tool of the medical detective. It is the branch of science that studies the patterns, causes, and effects of health and disease conditions in defined populations. The worldwide symbol of field epidemiologists is the "hole in the sole," evidence that we have worn out our shoes tracking down vital clues.

Until recently, courses in epidemiology were usually available only in advanced degree programs of medicine and public health. Now, fortunately, such courses are part of a growing number of American universities' undergraduate programs in public health.

Because public health or population health is not well understood by the American public, I wrote these stories to help readers better understand and value the public health system that exists for the protection of the nation's health and for the prevention of disease and injury. My purpose also was to show the work of medical detectives as interesting, often fascinating, and personally rewarding, and to encourage young scientists to enter a field where dedication to improving the lives of others has its own reward.

For this book, I tried to follow the format of the Sherlock Holmes stories by focusing on "cases" in which I was part of the investigation. Unlike Mr. Holmes, however, I was never the most important leader. A medical detective has a small part in a team effort, usually a very large team. Perhaps millions participated in the worldwide smallpox eradication effort, and certainly the investigation of the AIDS epidemic involved hundreds of thousands of scientists and public health and healthcare workers around the world.

Another difference between Sherlock Holmes's stories and those of medical detectives is that Holmes almost always solved the mystery. After more than thirty years of "investigation" of the AIDS epidemic, the control of this infection is still a mystery. We have neither an effective vaccine nor a cure.

Nor have we "solved" the Ebola epidemic, ongoing in West Africa since 2014. The Ebola virus is especially worrisome because of its relative ease of transmission after exposure and its high mortality rate. One can only be in awe of the many dedicated workers who have volunteered to serve in such a dangerous environment. Not the least of these are the medical detectives who collect clues, analyze data, investigate suspected cases, and carry out their public health mission.

ONE

My First Outbreak Investigation

IT WAS the evening of August 9, 1974. I was sitting at a bar in Atlanta, Georgia, watching President Richard M. Nixon resign from office. My rented, furnished apartment was nearby, but it had no television, and I did not want to miss seeing this historic event.

Also nearby was the Centers for Disease Control (CDC),* the only federal agency with headquarters outside of the Washington, DC, area, and my new employer of several weeks. Since the first week of July, I had been taking an intensive course in epidemiology and biostatistics. The course was my official introduction to the Epidemic Intelligence Service (EIS), a two-year epidemiology training program for which CDC was justifiably famous. I was lucky enough to be among the forty-five EIS officers, as we were called, selected for the EIS class of 1974. Of the thirty-nine physicians in the class, I was the only woman. In the early seventies, less than 10 percent of medical graduates in the United States were women. In the internal medicine training program that I had just completed, I was the only woman.

EIS officers are on call twenty-four hours a day to respond to requests for CDC assistance in the investigation of disease out-

---

*In 1974, CDC was actually called the Center for Disease Control. Since that time, the CDC acronym has been kept, but the official name of the agency has changed to the Centers for Disease Control and, finally, to the Centers for Disease Control and Prevention.

breaks or other public health emergencies. Each officer is matched either with a branch or program at CDC or with field stations, such as state or local health departments. I was matched with the Hospital Infections Program at CDC.

I did not have to wait long for my first outbreak. On August 28, my supervisor, Dr. Walter Stamm, came to my office and told me that a branch of the military had called CDC to request help with an outbreak of *Pseudomonas* sepsis (a bacterial blood infection) in the intensive care unit (ICU) of a large military hospital. As far as anyone could remember, this was the first time that the military had requested help from CDC. I had been chosen to go, and I was told it was to be kept confidential. Arrangements were being made for my travel orders and flights while I spoke with Dr. Stamm and other colleagues, who gave me information about the organism causing the outbreak and other briefing materials. Then I was told to go home, pack a bag, and be ready to leave on a plane later that afternoon.

In those days, airport security was minimal, and one could just enter the airport and proceed to a flight without being subject to screening. Upon arriving at the airport, I ran directly to the gate with my paper ticket and was the last passenger to get on the flight.

During the flight I reviewed my orders. I was a member of the Commissioned Corps of the Public Health Service, a uniformed service presided over by the US surgeon general. The corps headquarters in Washington issued our orders. Although a uniformed service, CDC officers at that time were exempt from wearing uniforms. (I believe one reason was to keep EIS officers relatively anonymous when they were investigating outbreaks.) So I was wearing plain clothes on the flight.

When the plane was preparing to descend, the pilot announced that landing would be delayed because horses had escaped from a nearby ranch and were on the airport runway. A small plane had collided with some of the horses, and we could not land until the runway was clear. We circled for more than two hours. Finally, we landed sometime after midnight.

A weary military escort team was waiting for me with a sign that read "Dr. Guinan, CDC." I walked up to the uniformed four men and one woman and identified myself. The men were clearly shocked that "Dr. Guinan" was a woman, and they were apologetic. They had not known that "CDC was sending a woman."

The everyday dress code for EIS officers was casual at CDC; some even wore jeans and t-shirts to work. Because I had had no time to change, I was wearing what I had worn to work that morning—a long-sleeved plaid shirt, black slacks, and Earth shoes, comfortable, sensible shoes made in Sweden that had heels lower than soles, supposedly good for the back and spine (they weren't). I wore no makeup, and my hair was tied behind my head in a long braid, a hairstyle that my colleagues told me gave me the appearance of being a "hippie." (Hippies were associated with the peace movement and the anti–Vietnam War marches that had torn the country apart. President Nixon had ended the war only a year earlier.) I wondered whether I should have given more thought to what I wore.

The uniformed officers took me to the base where the hospital was located. The base commander had closed the operating room and had called an "all-hands" meeting of healthcare personnel for the next day at 7:00 a.m., and I was asked to attend. The female member of the escort team was the hospital infection control nurse, Sarah,* one of a small number of woman officers at the hospital. She had arranged for me to stay off base in her home during my investigation. This was a great advantage for me: I did not have to worry about a place to stay, and I also had the infection control nurse as an

---

* Because of the confidentiality agreement, I have not identified the military base, the state, or the names of personnel involved except the first name of this infection control nurse.

ally in the investigation. Sarah told me that she was the only member of the escort team who knew beforehand that I was a woman, and she had not told the others. We laughed about their reaction.

The next morning I arrived for the meeting at the auditorium, which was packed with well over a hundred uniformed personnel. I sat in the back and noted that I was the only person not in uniform. The base commander was the speaker. He discussed the hospital's serious situation. It had eight cases of *Pseudomonas* blood infection in patients in the ICU, and the surgical suite had been closed, except for emergencies. Although the base commander did not mention it, many of the people who were ill were high-ranking officers. In fact, CDC had advised me before I left that one of the possibilities that the staff on the base were entertaining was that the blood had been deliberately contaminated with the *Pseudomonas* organism. Was someone trying to kill the officers? This concern was one of the main reasons that the investigation was to be kept confidential.

The base commander reinforced the seriousness of the situation by stating that it was the "first time in history" that a military hospital had called in an outside agency for assistance in an outbreak investigation. Furthermore, he said, "Let me tell you how fast CDC works. Yesterday we called CDC, and before 7 p.m. their expert was on his way here, and he is in the audience right now. Will he please stand up?"

I didn't. I did not want to embarrass either the base commander or myself. (Had someone deliberately not told him that I was a woman?) After looking around and seeing no one standing, the base commander finished his talk by asking for cooperation in the continuing investigation and stating that the operating room (OR) would remain closed until the source of the contamination was identified and eliminated.

After the meeting, I was introduced to the commander, who thanked me for coming. Then Sarah introduced me to the director of the infectious diseases unit and to many of the surgeons, nurses, and other personnel involved in the care of these case-patients.* The most frequent question I was asked was how long I had worked at CDC. Each time I answered "a while." I was worried about CDC's and my credibility if word spread that the CDC expert was not only a woman but also one who had been working at CDC for only several weeks.

Before my arrival, the hospital infection control team, led by Sarah, had undertaken an intensive investigation to find the source of the contamination of the patients' blood. Over the next several days, I reviewed all the data that they had collected. I interviewed a number of the surgeons and nurses to get their opinions on what was causing the blood contamination. Some expressed concern that the OR environment might be contaminated. I asked for a tour of the now-closed OR, where most believed the blood contamination had occurred.

It was in a very old building, and the OR was large, with extraordinarily high ceilings. The cleaning crew described how they cleaned the OR after each surgery and pointed out that the ceiling and the highest part of the walls near the ceiling were not cleaned daily. The crew also saw flies occasionally buzzing close to the ceiling and indicated that the flies were quite difficult to eliminate. The cleaning crew asked for my opinion on whether these could be factors. I did not know, so I wrote in my notes to do a review of the literature on infectious outbreaks in ORs. Were any due to environmental contamination?

We reviewed blood bank procedures. All coronary bypass patients receive multiple blood transfusions. I was guided through the process of how the heart-lung bypass machine was connected to

---

*"Case-patient" is a term epidemiologists use to distinguish patients with a case of the disease under study from all other patients in a given facility.

the patient and was told how many units of blood were used on average for each patient undergoing coronary artery bypass surgery. After the first few cases of sepsis had occurred, Sarah had begun culturing the blood from the blood bank before its use in the patients. All these cultures were negative. Her investigation found no evidence that the blood was contaminated before use.

Working in the office I was provided at the hospital, I reviewed the medical records of each case. The case definition we used was "a patient in the intensive care unit with a blood culture positive for *Pseudomonas aeruginosa*," that is, a case-patient, as opposed to the other patients in the ICU. Many of the case-patients, who had been treated with two intravenous antibiotics for which the organism was susceptible, had remained culture positive two to five days after the onset of treatment, which was very unusual. Either the organism was being reintroduced to the bloodstream or the antibiotics were not effective (even though laboratory testing showed the organism was susceptible). The great fear was that the organism would become resistant to these antibiotics. There were no other antibiotics that were effective against *Pseudomonas* at that time.

Several of the earlier case-patients who had been transferred out of the ICU had negative blood cultures and were doing well. This was a clue. I again reviewed the medical records of each case and tracked the chronology of the positive blood cultures. All case-patients had become culture positive in the ICU and culture negative after discharge from the ICU. Could it be that something or someone in the ICU was contaminating the case-patients' blood?

I shared my findings with Sarah. She told me that she had also recognized this pattern. The ICU was brand-new, having opened only a few months before my arrival. The director and staff were proud of the survival rate of the patients. Compared to the OR, the ICU was state-of-the-art and had all of the latest technical equipment. Sarah said that no one wanted to hear that this beautiful new

ICU could be the place where contamination of patients' blood was occurring.

Only two case-patients remained in the ICU. One was a 23-year-old man who had crashed his motorcycle and had multiple injuries, including a crushed chest with collapse of both lungs. He was unconscious, on a ventilator, and in critical condition. Two days after entering the ICU, he had developed a fever. Blood cultures were drawn and found to be positive for the *Pseudomonas* organism. He had not been in the OR nor had he received blood transfusions. These were the next clues. The contamination had to be occurring in the ICU because that was the only place he had been since admission. And this patient was still blood-culture positive. His blood cultures were continually positive during the week of antibiotic treatment.

I again reviewed his medical chart. During Sarah's systematic investigation, she had cultured many environmental areas in the ICU, which included specialized equipment that attached patients to the monitoring screens. Two of the transducers that were connected to the many tubes in this critically ill patient had been found to be culture positive for *Pseudomonas*.

A transducer is a device that converts energy from one form to another. For example, in one artery in the patient's arm, there was a tiny tube called a catheter, which was attached to a larger tube filled with a saline solution. This tube was attached to a transducer, which converted the pressure signal from the artery to an electrical signal, which appeared on the monitor as a blood pressure reading. This connection provided continuous monitoring of the patient's blood pressure. If the blood pressure reading moved out of the desired range, an alarm would alert ICU personnel to examine the patient and to institute procedures to stabilize it. If not corrected within minutes, a precipitous drop in blood pressure in this critically ill patient would likely result in severe brain damage or death. The motorcyclist was being monitored from two additional sites, one in the heart and one in the pulmonary system; both of these sites were also connected to transducers.

I spoke to Sarah about these findings. She said she had informed the ICU director about the contaminated transducers. But because of a shortage of transducers in the unit, there were none to replace the contaminated ones, and the director thought that the patient might die if his vital signs were not continuously monitored and stabilized. So he had not removed them. He was the director of the unit and outranked Sarah, so he essentially had the last word.

I asked to speak with the ICU director. I told him that I believed that the transducers were the source of the patient's blood contamination. He told me he felt that because nothing was flushed into the patient from the transducer lines, they were unlikely to be the source of the contamination. He pointed out that there was almost two feet of tubing between the transducer and the patient's blood, and it would be close to impossible for the bacteria to get from the transducer to the patient's blood. I told him that I believed that the patient might die of sepsis if the transducers were not removed. He said that the patient would likely die if the transducers *were* removed.

I called Walt Stamm at CDC for assistance. He agreed that the transducers were the likely source of the problem. He connected us with a CDC microbiologist who was an expert in *Pseudomonas* organisms. The three of us discussed the situation. I noted the two feet of tubing between the transducer and the patient's blood and the director's disbelief that the organisms could enter the bloodstream from that distance.

The microbiologist was exasperated. "*Pseudomonas* can swim!" he said. "I don't know how fast they can swim, but they are great swimmers."

I told him that the patient became culture positive within two days of entering the ICU.

"Then it takes two days for *Pseudomonas* organisms to swim down that two feet of saline solution," he said. "Or even less, since the blood was first cultured on the second day, when the patient developed a fever. The *Pseudomonas* might have been down there within a few hours. We don't know."

Dr. Stamm and the microbiologist agreed that I should again ask that the transducers be removed. If they weren't, I should consider going to a higher authority. I asked Sarah if I could speak to the director again. She made the request. We were told he would not be available until the next day.

I became very concerned. Sarah and I reviewed how the transducers were sterilized. We found out that because of a large caseload in the ICU, there were insufficient transducers for all patients. As a result, the usual sterilization process was being bypassed. The transducers had not been sterilized according to the manufacturer's directions. Instead of being put in an autoclave, a pressure chamber used to sterilize materials (a process that took several hours), the transducers that were taken from infected patients were cleaned with multiple flushes of an iodine antiseptic solution and then re-used on another patient. The motorcyclist had received at least one of these transducers.

I told Sarah what CDC had recommended and that *Pseudomonas* organisms could swim, which would essentially invalidate the ICU director's assumptions. I asked her to convey, again, my request to speak with him and that she convey that the request was urgent.

When we were connected by telephone later that day, the ICU director told me that he could not remove the transducers because the patient would die and that I would be responsible for the patient's death.

I told Sarah his response and asked her who would be the higher authority to whom I should appeal. She left me alone in my office.

Some time later, she returned with the chief of infectious diseases, the ICU director, and the commander of the base.

I explained the reasoning and asked that the contaminated transducers be removed. I explained that the blood cultures continued to be positive, and now the organism was beginning to show some resistance to the antibiotics. The ICU director refused. The base commander, who outranked the ICU director, ordered him to remove the transducers. It was by now late in the evening. By the time Sarah and I left for her home, she told me that the transducers and all the attached tubing that entered the patient's body had been removed.

I did not sleep well that night. I was fearful of the patient's status. The next morning, the patient was in the same condition—no better or worse. Blood cultures were drawn. Again I reviewed the medical charts of all the cases. All of the case-patients except the motorcyclist had been transferred out of the ICU. All their blood cultures were now negative.

The next day, the blood cultures of the motorcyclist were negative, and he was beginning to regain consciousness. Repeat cultures the following day were also negative, and his fever was gone.

I called CDC, and Dr. Stamm told me to come home. He said that the base commander had called him earlier, told him I had solved the problem, and praised me as being a cross between "Einstein and Wonder Woman."

Going over the outbreak on my flight home, it was clear to me that *I* had not solved the problem. Sarah and her team had. They had amassed all the evidence, evidence that had convinced me of the source of the problem. Then the backup professional staff at CDC had guided me to do what apparently was the right thing.

And I was greatly relieved that the base commander was not disappointed that CDC had sent a woman.

TWO

Something to Believe In

OPERATION SMALLPOX ZERO

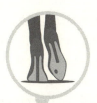

WHEN asked as a child what I wanted to be when I grew up, I used to reply "a plumber or a doctor." Laughter was the usual response, as neither was a likely profession for a woman at the time. Although it was a circuitous route, I did finally find my way to becoming a physician and to a satisfying career in public health.

FROM COLLEGE TO CHICLETS

I grew up in New York City, the third of five children of Irish immigrant parents, who met on the ship bringing them to America in 1928. They had left their families and political oppression to find freedom and opportunity not available to them in Ireland. Because as children they had been needed to work the farms, they had no more than three or four years of formal grade-school education. Despite the difficult years of the Great Depression that followed their arrival, my parents warmly embraced their new country. They often told us (especially if we complained) how blessed we were to be born in the greatest country in the world with the freedom to follow our dreams.

My parents made it clear to us that we were going to go to college. We had no idea how that would happen, but we accepted college as a given and never questioned it. My father worked in the New York subway system, and my mother was a homemaker. I was a teenager when my father died suddenly. We children all found jobs and worked our way through high school and college. My mother found work as a salesperson in a department store during the Christmas season and eventually held a full-time job there.

Fortunately, I was accepted into Hunter College of the City University of New York. Not only was there no tuition for students who maintained the necessary grades, but Hunter also provided textbooks for all my courses for only $20 per semester. My mother told me I had to find a profession with which I could support myself "and stand on my own two feet." I started out majoring in Greek and Latin studies. After I completed a first-year chemistry course, the professor asked to meet with me. Because I didn't yet know my grade, I thought perhaps I had not done well on the final exam. But the professor told me that I had done very well, that I was good in chemistry, and that I should consider making it my major. It was such a surprise to me that I said I didn't think so. He urged me to take another chemistry course to see how I would do. Thinking about my mother's advice, I decided that perhaps I could better support myself as a chemist than as a Greek and Latin scholar, so I took the next-level chemistry course, did well, and became a chemistry major.

By the time I graduated from college, I knew that I wanted to be a physician, but at the time women were rarely admitted to medical school. Besides, one criterion for admission was having the money to pay for it. I did not, and scholarships were not available.

So I started searching for a job as a chemist. The *New York Times* want ads were segregated by gender back then, and there was never an ad for a chemist in the female listings. Sometimes I applied for the jobs listed in the male ads, but doing so was both humiliating and unsuccessful. Finally, I found a position in a chewing gum factory for the American Chicle Division of Warner-Lambert Pharmaceutical Company in Queens, New York. The company made Chiclets, Trident, Black Jack, and all sorts of chewing gum. My job was to help develop chewing gum with new flavors. My new position greatly amused my friends and family. I thought it paid well until I found out that I was paid considerably less than my male peers.

This realization moved me to apply to graduate schools for an advanced degree in chemistry. More often than not, I would receive a one-page reply saying either that the program did not accept women or that it did not provide female students with financial assistance.

THE SPACE PROGRAM

Just as I was feeling frustrated with a lack of opportunities to attend graduate school, the space program opened up. President John F. Kennedy announced in 1961 that within the decade he wanted the United States to put a man on the moon and bring him back safely. The need for scientists to participate in the space program was enormous. Federal money was allocated to support students to get advanced degrees in science to help fill the program's need. In his inaugural address, President Kennedy had said, "And so, my fellow Americans: ask not what your country can do for you—ask what you can do for your country."

Two years later, I was sitting in my laboratory tasting a sample of a new flavored gum that I had submitted for production. A colleague entered the lab and told me that President Kennedy had been shot. Profoundly affected by the news of his death, I decided that I would try to become an astronaut.

I found an ad in a science journal from the University of Texas Medical Branch (UTMB), in Galveston, offering stipends for doctoral students. I found out that UTMB was located close to Clear Lake City, the home of the National Aeronautics and Space Administration (NASA). I applied to the doctoral program in physiology and within two weeks received a reply from the chair of the department that I had been accepted. But the letter did not mention financial support. I wrote back, asking if a graduate assistantship were available. I received my letter back with a handwritten note at the bottom that said, "We are holding one for you," signed Mason Guest, PhD. This was one of the great thrills of my life.

I arrived in Galveston not knowing anyone there. Because it was such a radical idea, I did not reveal my ambition to be an astronaut. The program was wonderful. On occasion, an astronaut who had been in space (such as Alan Shepard, John Glenn, or Scott Carpenter) would lecture in our class and tell us stories about his experiences. It was a heady, exciting time for a scientist, and I loved it. About two years into the program, I told Dr. Guest, who was by then my mentor, that I wanted to be an astronaut. He advised me that it would be difficult and that I should get my degree before I let this be known because he thought I might be subject to ridicule.

Just before completing my doctorate, I attended an aviation and space medicine class at NASA with about ten other students. On the last day, the teacher distributed a form that asked whether we met the medical and physical requirements for acceptance into the astronaut program. I was the only woman in the class and also the only one who fulfilled the requirements because of my good health, height, weight, and 20/20 vision. (In the 1960s, astronauts had to fit into a small capsule inside the spacecraft, so height and weight were of great importance.) Despite having the preliminary qualifications, I was not asked to apply for the astronaut program.

I knew it was unlikely that I would actually be chosen to be an astronaut because there was tremendous competition. By then, it was 1968, when preparations for the moon landing were in full swing. Command central in Houston was the control center for all moon-landing activities. When I read in a newspaper article that women were not permitted into command central, not even to bring coffee, "because they might distract the men," I knew that there was little chance a woman would become an astronaut within the next few years.*

Dr. Guest helped me to get a postdoctoral fellowship at the National Institutes of Health (NIH) in Bethesda, Maryland, studying aspects of blood coagulation, which had been the subject of my dissertation. The Vietnam War was under way, and I took the place of man who had been drafted. Most positions at NIH required an MD, so I did not envision a future there. Then a mentor at NIH suggested that I fix that and go to medical school—my first dream, of so many years before.

And so I did. I was accepted to Johns Hopkins School of Medicine, where I found, surprisingly, that 10 percent of students were women—a requirement of a donor, Mary Elizabeth Garrett. The faculty were supportive of my getting experiences that were not part of the academic curriculum. I applied for a US government fellowship to study tropical diseases for a semester and was sent to Guadalajara, Mexico. There I spent several weeks seeing patients at a leprosy clinic and then was assigned to the Hospital Civil, where during a polio outbreak I saw my first cases of polio, including several affected children in iron lungs. This amazing experience sparked my interest in infectious diseases.

I graduated in 1972. The medical degree, together with my doctorate in physiology in the area of blood coagulation, would prepare me for a career as a hematologist/oncologist, most likely in academic medicine. That was the plan.

---

*I didn't make it to space, but gum from my first chemist job did! It was a point of pride at American Chicle that Trident chewing gum was selected as the gum that the first astronauts would take to space.

OPERATION SMALLPOX ZERO

It was in 1971, in my last year of medical school, when I first heard of the plan to eliminate the dreaded disease smallpox from the world.

The United States was still engaged in the Vietnam War, and massive national protests against it were growing. When the United States bombed Cambodia in 1970, expanding the war, an antiwar protest by Kent State University students was answered by Ohio National Guard troops. Four unarmed students were shot and killed, and nine others were wounded. It was difficult to believe—our government killing unarmed student protesters on a college campus!

The country was emerging from the chaotic 1960s, when President John F. Kennedy, Senator Robert Kennedy, and civil rights leader Dr. Martin Luther King Jr. were killed by assassins' bullets. The United States and the Soviet Union were entrenched in the Cold War, and multitudes were protesting the ongoing Vietnam War.

During my medical residency, I was beginning to have second thoughts about a career in academic medicine. The Smallpox Eradication Program again came to my attention, this time in a magazine article that described the implementation of the program and the participation of CDC. That federal agency was sending volunteers to the World Health Organization (WHO), which was leading the eradication program. I was captivated by the idea that a group of idealists had laid out a plan to eradicate smallpox from the world and that our government was a partner. If this mission worked, it would be the first time in history that a human disease was eliminated by the design of humans. Smallpox, a horrible disease feared by civilizations from earliest recorded history, would then be gone. It was an exhilarating idea.

I applied to CDC's Epidemic Intelligence Service (EIS), a two-year program that trained participants in the control of disease outbreaks (and much more, I was to find out). I was accepted into the class of 1974, which began in July. I knew next to nothing about epidemiology and was never interested in a career in public health. But the EIS was my route to joining the smallpox eradication effort.

I was assigned to the Hospital Infections Program in Atlanta and began the work of an EIS officer. Every week at the mandatory EIS officers' conference, there would be a call for volunteers for the Smallpox Eradication Program in India. I applied twice but was not selected; I was told that WHO was not accepting women into the program. I protested to the director of the EIS program, Philip Brachman, MD, who told me that it was not WHO but India that was not accepting women. I pointed out that the prime minister of India, Indira Gandhi, was a woman and asked whether she knew about this. I asked to speak to someone at WHO or in India to plead my case. Dr. Brachman said he would look into it. The next week, I was accepted. I was ecstatic.

On December 31, 1974, I joined ten physician volunteers in Delhi for a training course given by Bill Foege, MD, the director of the eradication program in India, and Dr. Nicole Grasset, a Swiss-French medical virologist-epidemiologist who directed the regional WHO office. We learned about the search (surveillance)-and-containment strategy for smallpox that Bill had begun in Africa. (This strategy, which Bill had used to great success in Africa, was conceived because of a smallpox vaccine shortage there. Basically, instead of vaccinating everyone—that is, mass vaccination—smallpox teams found smallpox patients, isolated them, and vaccinated their contacts and every unvaccinated person within a ten-mile radius.) This strategy was so successful that Bill continued to use and evaluate the method. Although there were a number of naysayers who did not believe that the method would work in India, Bill had promoted it, rather than mass vaccination, as the primary approach for eradicating the disease in that country. During his first year in India, the results were so impressive that one could actually imagine that smallpox would be eradicated.

Our group of volunteers finished our training in early January 1975 and reported to our assigned programs just at the start of Operation Smallpox Zero. By that time the eradication program was remarkably successful, and there was a great deal of optimism. Smallpox outbreaks were still occurring, but in only two states in India, in remote parts of Uttar Pradash (UP) and Bihar, in northeastern India close to Nepal. I was one of three sent to UP. Accompanying me were Walt Orenstein, MD, a fellow EIS officer, and J. Michael McGinnis, MD, from the Office on International Health in Washington, DC. We were met at the airport in the capital city, Lucknow, by Don Francis, MD, the director of the program in UP. When Don saw us, he said, "What am I going to do with three Americans?" It was the time of the Cold War, and it was an extremely sensitive issue that all units have approximately equal representations of American and Soviet epidemiologists. Three Americans would upset the balance in UP.

We joined a team of about twenty epidemiologists assigned to different areas to do surveillance and containment. Each of us was allocated various supplies and staff, including vaccine and bifurcated needles, sleeping bags, a jeep with driver, and a paramedical assistant, who served as navigator, cook, interpreter, procurer of food, and general all-around invaluable aide.

Our job was to go to our assigned area, find persons infected with smallpox (patients), immediately immunize all contacts of the patients, and then surround them with a ring of immunity, that is, the ten-mile radius of a patient's village. We were to quarantine patients until the infection was no longer communicable, and vaccinate everyone within the prescribed radius. Smallpox spreads only from person to person. If you interrupt the chain of transmission with an immunized population, the virus has no place to go.

I had been assigned to Kanpur, which had been declared smallpox-free, and I would just be doing surveillance activities unless we found a smallpox case. Shafi, my paramedical assistant, and I would be going from village to village to show pictures of children with smallpox, promising a reward of 10 rupees for anyone who led us to a case.

But fate intervened. A few days before our arrival in UP, there were unconfirmed reports of smallpox cases in another area that had also been declared smallpox-free. Dr. Francis told me he was going to send me not to Kanpur but to Rampur Matras to determine whether the reported cases were actually smallpox. It was an amazing experience for me—having never seen a case of small-pox—to be the decision maker. But following the protocol we learned in Delhi, I examined the patient, a young Brahmin man, and declared he had smallpox.

The die was cast. I would be in Rampur Matras for the next two months, overseeing the vaccination program in the villages surrounding the case. The patient's elders had brought him to a prostitute for his first sexual experience, which resulted in his contracting smallpox. The issue was quite sensitive, and the family refused to reveal the location of the prostitute.

Despite the caste system's being banned in India, it was still intact in rural areas, and Brahmins were a high caste. Those from lower castes were not to touch a Brahmin. In order to get a sample of the pustules of the patient to send to Delhi for confirmation of smallpox, someone had to touch the young man. The father finally permitted me to take the sample. Shafi later told me it was because of my light skin color; lower castes were associated with dark skin.

I had only the tiniest of maps, and it was difficult to determine the ten-mile radius, so we just began vaccinating in the adjacent villages. Shafi started the process by putting out a call for local government vaccinators. How all this worked without any kind of telephone contact was always a mystery to me. But vaccinators arrived within a day.

They would be paid a good stipend for their work, over and above their regular pay. Shafi took care of the ledger, registering the vaccinators and keeping track of the days they worked. At the end of each week, I had to pay them. WHO had issued all epidemiologists a series of checks in rupees that could be cashed at local banks. Shafi and the driver (who liked to be called "Driver," rather than his given name) always knew how to find the local bank, even in the most remote area. The first week we hired over thirty vaccinators. So I cashed several hundred rupees' worth of checks and got small bills of 1, 5, and 10 rupees. I put the money in a travel belt, which I had brought with me from home. I kept the money belt under my shirt above my abdomen, where it wouldn't be obvious. We followed this routine every week for two months. Sometimes I had more money than the belt could hold, and I would put the excess in the pockets of my pants.

If we came back from the bank after dark, we worried about roadblocks, and the possibility that thieves could stop us and take our money. Shafi prepared me in advance for a potential roadblock. He said my light skin would be a giveaway that I was a foreigner and would be more likely to have money. So I bought a large woolen shawl that covered my head and whole upper body, including my hands. Whenever we drove at night, I wore this shawl. In the months I was there, we were stopped only once at a roadblock. I was under the shawl, and I could not see nor understand the conversation. I did not move. Shafi was successful in getting us past the roadblock without incident.

Our work was often complicated by the local populace's lack of understanding of the program or by logistical problems. Cultural issues arose on a daily basis. Driver was Hindu; he spoke only Hindi. My assistant, Shafi, was Muslim; he spoke Urdu, Hindi, and English. I did not speak Hindi or Urdu, but I did learn to read the Hindi symbols so that I could read road signs. (Driver was unable to read, so I would phonetically sound out the symbols so he knew which way to go.)

I was a woman traveling with two men who were not my family members, an extremely unusual occurrence in Indian culture. This area of UP was 99 percent illiterate. Most of the people in the area had never seen a foreigner nor even heard of America. They did not have a concept of another country or language and thus could not understand why I did not understand them. (Occasionally, when Shafi was asked where I was from, he would say, "Oh, she's from Lucknow.")

I was a source of great curiosity. I had anticipated some of this and had dyed my blond hair black before I left the United States so that I wouldn't be too conspicuous. I had had several outfits made for me in Lucknow—wide pants with pockets and long shirts, or *Kurtas*, much like what the Muslim women wore. Indian women wore saris, and I could usually distinguish whether we were in a Muslim or Hindu village by the women's clothing.

The women welcomed me. In fact, often in a Muslim village the women would insist I come into their huts because they could not come out. Staying inside was part of their practice. Shafi would not be allowed in. In the hut, I used a kind of sign language with the women, and I learned a lot—that most of the women were pregnant, for example, and that they had babies every year. When we were vaccinating, if I saw a child of about one year old in a hut, I would look around for a baby; somewhere, perhaps hidden in a blanket, there was almost always another baby. The women in turn would pat my abdomen and ask where *my* babies were. While I was there, several babies were born and named America.

I stayed in mud huts or camped out in the various villages we visited. It was very cold. I thought India would be extremely hot, but UP is in the north, and it was cold. When I arrived at the Delhi airport, it was 3 degrees Celsius (37 degrees Fahrenheit), and I did not have warm clothes. So I had a quilt made in Lucknow, which I used both as a shawl and as a blanket for warmth.

And there were rats. They occasionally came into my hut at night, which terrified me. One morning, I found one in my purse. When I told Driver, he just opened the purse and let the rat out. Indians respected life and tried not to kill anything.

Shafi had a small, oil-heated stove on which he cooked our meals. He and Driver ate with their fingers. I never managed to do this, but Shafi, as usual, was prepared. He brought with him an old spoon that I used. Driver's Hindu beliefs forbade him to eat out of the same plate as Shafi and me. Because we had only one plate, we would find leaves that Driver could use as a plate.

One day, while crossing one of the numerous rivers intersecting the villages, I rolled up my pants above my knees, took off my shoes, and waded across. No one was there when I started across, but about fifty villagers had gathered by the time I got to the other side. All appeared to be in a state of shock, staring at me in complete silence. To my immense embarrassment, I remembered that in this cultural setting a woman showing her legs was highly inappropriate. The story spread, although I don't know how, and months later, when I returned to WHO headquarters in Delhi, I received considerable ribbing about it.

It could take weeks for the results from the smallpox lab, so during the remainder of my time in India, I continued working as if all the suspect cases we found were truly smallpox. We hired family members to care for the patient (so they would not leave the hut), and we hired three vaccinators to guard each hut. They worked eight-hour shifts. Anybody who went in the hut had to be vaccinated. We returned for surprise inspections to make sure that a guard was on duty.

I kept on this way—culturing, sending off the samples, hiring vaccinators—and learned something the first few weeks of vaccinating. If we went to a village, talked to its leader, and said we wanted to vaccinate everyone, we found that we were often missing people. So we came up with a different strategy. We would first take a census of the village, writing down everyone's name and approximate age. Taking a census implied that resources might be coming, so the people were very cooperative. The next day we vaccinated everyone on the list.

About this time, Don Francis came from Lucknow to visit me. He was worried.

"Listen," he said, "this place was declared free of smallpox and you are sending off all of these samples saying there's smallpox. Are you sure?"

"As sure as I can be," I answered.

"Are you *sure*?" he repeated. "Because you're causing a political problem for the public health leader of the area who has declared it free of smallpox." The cultures eventually all came back positive.

While Don was there, he also checked the vaccination rates in the villages where we had finished vaccinating. He would walk through the village asking the children to show him their smallpox vaccination. He did not find a single unvaccinated child.

We did our work and once a month went to Lucknow for a meeting. I would check into my hotel the night before the meeting and have my first bath in a month, get my laundry done, and then eat dinner with my colleagues.

Dr. Foege would come up from Delhi for this session, and each of us would present our data on the number of outbreaks we had found and how we had contained them. Bill would share the results from Bihar. A little competition developed among us concerning whether Bihar or UP would reach Smallpox Zero first. Each month, the outbreaks continued to go down dramatically. It was apparent we were approaching the goal of zero smallpox cases. Dr. Foege's book, *House on Fire* (1), captures the excitement of those days and gives an extensive account of the worldwide smallpox eradication effort.

At the monthly meetings, Walt Orenstein and I would have dinner together. We are both from New York, and we would share stories about how our team would not understand our humor. We would say something we thought was funny, and they would stare at us blankly. We had lots of laughs about this, and we became life-long friends.

When the smallpox workers were at the hotel in Lucknow, vendors would come and peddle their wares. A particular rug dealer, who was called the "rug walla," would target Walt and me. The rug walla would come to the hotel with his assistant, who was laden with rugs. He would stand outside the window of the restaurant where we were eating and have his assistant hold up one of at least five or six rugs. We would shake our heads yes or no, depending on whether we liked each one. Every month he came and found us, and eventually the rug walla's persistence paid off. Walt and I both bought a number of rugs and had them sent back to the States.

Walt and I also exchanged information about successful techniques to be used in the field. One was an approach of another colleague, who found unvaccinated children by offering candy. We brought a large quantity of paper-covered toffees back with us to the field. When we walked through the villages, we would ask the children to show us their smallpox vaccination scars. If they had one, we gave them a toffee. If they didn't, we first vaccinated them and then gave them a toffee. This approach proved very successful. When children saw us coming, they would run to us to get the toffee.

After we finished the work in Rampur Matras, I was assigned to Kanpur, which was still smallpox free. I continued the surveillance process. By now the reward was 100 rupees, and I think that it reached 1,000 rupees before the end of the campaign. Unfortunately, my request to CDC to stay in India until the goal of zero cases was reached was denied. I left in April to return to my EIS officer position.

In May, Uttar Pradash was declared smallpox-free. It was one of the most exciting experiences of my life. The program had worked. And I was hooked. I decided to embark on a career in public health. I doubt I would have considered such a career had it not been for those idealists who conceived of the worldwide Smallpox Eradication Program, convinced world leaders that it was important, worked tenaciously to ensure the effort was successful, and gave people like me the chance to participate. I had found something to believe in.

THREE
A Gift of an Elephant

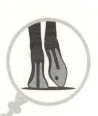

EARLY one morning in a small village in a remote area of India, our smallpox eradication team was preparing for the day's work when we spotted a fast-moving vehicle coming toward us on the dirt road. Although we had been in the area for about two or three weeks, I had never seen another vehicle there besides the Mahindra Mahindra jeep that was our main mode of transportation. The road was full of potholes after the rainy season, and dirt was swirling as the car bumped up and down.

All work stopped, and both villagers and smallpox workers watched in silence as the black, dirt-covered Mercedes pulled up beside me. A well-dressed, ebullient young man jumped out. He smiled, introduced himself in perfect English, and asked me what I was doing. After I explained that we were smallpox eradication workers, he said he had heard about us and thought it was a fantastic mission, and he wanted to help. Specifically, he had heard that we were having difficulty getting transportation back and forth across the rivers that intersected the smallpox-infected villages. This was true. The rivers were too deep for our jeep to traverse, and our means for crossing rivers were unpredictable.

The young man was called Raj Sahib (pronounced Raj Sob) by the locals, a term of deference used to refer to Indian men of middle and upper classes. As we talked, the whole village assembled around the Mercedes, keeping a respectful distance. Raj Sahib then announced, in English, that he was presenting me with an elephant. He said that the elephant swam and that she would solve our river-crossing problem.

Only the smallpox team members understood English, so they immediately translated what he said for the villagers. I thanked him profusely, but inwardly was a bit taken aback. I was unsure that we could actually *use* the elephant or what complications might ensue for an elephant under my care. I thought I would gracefully decline. Before I could do this, however, he pointed down the road, and we saw an elephant approaching in the distance. Raj Sahib said with a laugh, "I drive too fast and the elephant can't keep up."

The elephant moved slowly, with an almost bouncy walk. On her back was the driver, or *mahout*, wearing beautiful white clothes and a splendid turban. Raj Sahib insisted on showing me how the elephant swam, but the river was about a mile or so from the village. My assistant, Shafi, and I asked Raj Sahib to accompany us in the jeep, and we led the elephant and her driver to the river.

At the river, nearby villagers gathered to watch the process. The elephant's shoulders were approximately nine feet high. On her back was a large handmade saddle, made of what appeared to be hemp covered with a cloth. The mahout dismounted and unrolled a hemp ladder so I could mount. The ladder seemed flimsy and swung back and forth as I climbed up. The mahout had somehow gotten back up on the saddle and helped me on. It was neither an easy nor graceful mount. The elephant had light gray skin with pink patches, and I thought to myself, *Who would believe that I would be riding on a pink elephant?*

Before entering the river, Raj Sahib said that if the water were deep enough to go over the elephant's back, the elephant would pick me up in her trunk and hold me to keep me dry.

"No, no. Thank you, but no," I said. "I'm not doing that. It's okay if I get wet."

But the mahout did not speak English. So I asked Shafi to be sure to tell him that I did not want the elephant to pick me up in her trunk. After conversing back and forth with the mahout, Shafi told me that the driver had received orders from Raj Sahib for the elephant to pick me up if there were any danger of my getting wet. In such situations, the elephant usually picked up the mahout. I had a three-way conversation with Shafi, Raj Sahib, and the driver for several minutes, until Shafi assured me that everyone understood that, in the event of deep water, the elephant would pick up the mahout with her trunk and *not* me.

The elephant walked slowly into the water. Then suddenly the river deepened and she was swimming. She scooped up the mahout—but not me. We landed on the other side and then turned around and came back again, the elephant showing off her prowess. The demonstration was a complete success, and Raj Sahib was delighted. We returned in the jeep to the village, where Raj Sahib got into his Mercedes and drove away. I never saw him again.

And so my preparations began to include an elephant in the Smallpox Eradication Program. Before the elephant, our two possibilities to cross the river were by boat or by camel. We would pack everything into the jeep, drive to the river, and wait. Some days there was neither boat nor camel. Occasionally, a small boat, which was paddled by a standing man with a long stick, would appear. Shafi would negotiate with him to ferry us across. It would take several trips back and forth to get the two or three of us and all our supplies across. We would have to leave the jeep and driver at the river.

Once we had crossed the river, we had to walk 1 to 3 miles, carrying our sleeping bags, clothing, a cooking stove, any food that we might have purchased from local farmers, vaccine, needles, and the numerous supplies needed for taking culture samples and sending them to World Health Organization (WHO) headquarters in Delhi. We would go to a village with a suspected smallpox case and ask if anyone had seen a person with smallpox. Shafi would show a picture of a child with smallpox and tell the villagers who gathered around us that we would give a reward of 10 rupees to anyone who would lead us to a case. Any of the workers who found a smallpox-infected person would also receive 10 rupees. This was our surveillance system.

If we found nothing after a day's work, it could be difficult to return home. It was often too late to walk back to the river, and it was unlikely that we could find passage at night. So we would then look for food, and Shafi would cook dinner. Sometimes we found eggs and vegetables, and, rarely, Shafi would buy a chicken that he would kill and prepare for dinner. Food was scarce. The next morning we would walk back to the river and wait for another boat or camel.

Camels were more common than boatmen, but the camel drivers often refused to take us because the camels already had heavy loads. I disliked the camels because they were likely to bite, spit on, or kick strangers as well as to try to knock riders out of the saddle. I was bitten several times, mostly on my arms, where the camel could reach when it turned its head around while I was in the saddle. It was also difficult for a camel to carry more than two passengers (including the driver), which meant many more trips back and forth.

So the elephant was a dream addition to the team. She could accommodate many more people and supplies when crossing. And when we landed on the other side, the elephant took us to where we wanted to go, saving considerable time and energy. And we also had a guaranteed ride home anytime we wanted. We could leave our sleeping bags, clothing, and personal items in one village and leave a worker in charge. When we returned to the village in the evening, the worker would have found food for dinner and breakfast the next morning.

Each evening the elephant would return to her home. The next morning the elephant and driver would reappear. I arranged through

Shafi to pay the mahout a daily wage (for which he was delighted), but I paid nothing for the elephant. Elephants are a sign of wealth in India; because they eat so much, they are very expensive to keep.

We used the elephant for approximately three weeks and accomplished our objective of providing a 10-mile ring of immunity around each village with a smallpox patient much faster than anyone expected. When we left the area, I never got a chance to thank Raj Sahib. I knew no way to contact him.

WHO had to approve all expenditures by smallpox workers. The expense for the elephant driver was an unusual request to say the least, and I heard from colleagues that D. A. Henderson, MD, the director of the Smallpox Eradication Program stationed in Geneva, was fond of saying he had to justify "payments for Mary Guinan's elephant."

In 2010, I attended the celebration at CDC for the thirtieth anniversary of smallpox eradication. It was a wonderful affair, with memorable stories, many speeches, and catching up with many colleagues. When Dr. Henderson gave his talk, he again mentioned how he had to justify payments for my elephant. But after his address, I finally got to tell him, "D. A., the payments were for the elephant *driver*, not the elephant!" WHO couldn't afford an elephant.

FOUR

Dr. Herpes

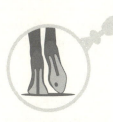

I DON'T think anyone grows up wanting to be a physician who specializes in sexually transmitted diseases (STDs). I certainly did not. And I suspect most of us who work in this area had dreams of different careers. My path to being an STD expert was circuitous, and I am very glad I stumbled upon it. I like to say that I have newscaster Dan Rather and Salt Lake City, Utah, to thank for steering me toward a career in STDs.

By 1976, I had left CDC and joined the infectious diseases training program at the University of Utah, where pioneering research on herpes simplex virus type 1 (HSV-1) infection was ongoing. HSV-1 is one of eight known herpesviruses that infect humans (table 1). It is the cause of cold sores.

Ever since I can remember, I have had frequent recurring bouts of cold sores around the lips and mouth. In elementary school, I was often sent home when I had cold sores, calling negative attention to my problem. Sun exposure, fever, dental appointments, and trauma to the mouth—any of these could trigger an outbreak, which could last one to two weeks. In college, as a last resort, I was treated with monthly smallpox vaccinations for twelve months to prevent recurrences. (This was a common, but unorthodox, treatment based on the erroneous idea that the vaccine would give a boost to the immune system and prevent recurrences. At that time, no effective treatment for HSV-1 infection existed, and well-meaning physi-

Table 1. Human herpesviruses

Human Herpesviruses	Alternative Names	Symptoms/Diseases	Site of Latency	Year Linked to Disease
Herpesvirus 1 HHV-1	Herpes simplex virus type 1 HSV-1	Cold sores; oral herpes; corneal infection, which can cause blindness; genital herpes, relatively rarely.	Trigeminal nerve cell body	First cultured in 1925
Herpesvirus 2 HHV-2	Herpes simplex virus type 2 HSV-2	Genital herpes; newborn infection; oral herpes, rarely.	Sacral nerve cell body	Recognized as sexually transmitted late 1960s
Herpesvirus 3 HHV-3	Varicella-zoster virus VZV	Chickenpox is first infection; zoster or shingles is recurrence.	Cranial and spinal nerve ganglia	First isolated in 1958
Herpesvirus 4 HHV-4	Epstein-Barr virus EBV	Mononucleosis. Also linked to Burkitt's lymphoma.	B lymphocytes	Linked to mononucleosis in 1968
Herpesvirus 5 HHV-5	Cytomegalovirus CMV	Sexually transmitted, usually without causing disease. Can cause severe disease in persons with compromised immune systems; mononucleosis, relatively rarely.	Suspected sites: monocytes, macrophages	Late 1950s
Herpesvirus 6 HHV-6		Causes roseola, high fever with rash in children.	Suspected site: CD4 lymphocytes	1988
Herpesvirus 7 HHV-7		Roseola, relatively rarely.	Suspected site: CD4 lymphocytes	1990
Herpesvirus 8 HHV-8	Kaposi's sarcoma virus	Kaposi's sarcoma.	Suspected site: B lymphocyte	1994

Note: All herpesviruses that infect humans have been renamed as human herpesvirus 1 through 8.

cians often resorted to unproven treatments.) On the bright side, although the treatment was ineffective for my cold sores, I never did get smallpox.

With my move to the University of Utah, I decided to focus my research and career on finding a treatment or cure for my lifelong affliction. And lifelong it is: once herpesviruses successfully invade a human host, they stay forever. There was a joke in those days that asked, "What is the difference between true love and herpes?" The answer: "Herpes lasts forever."

Infection with HSV-1 occurs throughout the world and is so common that by age 40 almost 90 percent of adults will have antibodies to it. It is a cunning virus, transmitted from person to person through close contact with the infected saliva. First exposure usually occurs in childhood, when the virus enters the mouth and infects cells of the skin or mucous membranes (epithelial cells). But it soon moves to a safe harbor in the cell body of a sensory nerve (trigeminal), where it remains in a so-called latent state. But it is not totally inactive; rather, it is silently lurking. The virus periodically reactivates just enough to move into the carrier's saliva, but it causes no symptoms, so the person does not know if or when it is there. I call this the virus's stealth strategy for jumping to a new host.

Only a small subset of infected persons has recurrences resulting in cold sores. The reason why is unknown; however, recent genetic-sequencing studies suggest that it may be due in part to different viral strains. In recurrences, the virus is activated by a trigger, which causes it to move out of the nerve cell and into the skin cells, where it causes cold sores on the lips or around the outside of the mouth. So a recurrence is an activation with symptoms.

With the University of Utah team, I conducted a double-blind, placebo-controlled study (the gold standard for determining drug efficacy) to determine the effectiveness of topical ether as a treatment for HSV-1. Preliminary reports had suggested that it might be an effective treatment (1). Ether penetrates the skin and destroys the lipid envelope of the virus, resulting in its destruction. It seemed like the perfect solution. To my immense disappointment, the treatment was completely ineffective (2).

Before publication, I presented the results at a national medical meeting in a special session on herpesviruses (3). Because of media interest, all eleven speakers were asked to attend a press briefing afterward. I don't remember the questions asked, but I noticed that a disproportionate number seemed to be addressed to me. (I thought it might be because I was the only woman speaker.) That evening, I turned on the *CBS Evening News* and was startled to see myself on the television screen, with Dan Rather saying, "Dr. Mary Guinan, an expert in genital herpes infections." And there I was, pointing to my lip.

I froze. I was stupefied. I had presented data and answered questions on *oral* herpes. Why did they think I was talking about *genital* herpes?

And it did not stop there. When I returned to Utah, two reporters—one from the local CBS affiliate and another from the local newspaper—met me at the airport. The university, which was delighted to discover it had an "expert in genital herpes," had given the reporters information on my flight arrival.

I explained that there was a misunderstanding, clarifying that my work was on oral herpes, not genital herpes. But the subsequent stories on the evening news and in the morning paper both reported I was studying genital herpes infection.

Soon thereafter I received numerous phone and letter requests for appointments from persons wanting help with genital herpes infection. At first, I did not respond. Then the dean's office called, saying that it had received several complaints about my lack of response to patient inquiries and asked that I please respond.

I felt like the lazy woodcutter in Moliere's comedy *The Doctor in Spite of Himself*, whose wife played a trick on him by telling high officials looking for a doctor that her husband was a wonderful physician. But she warned them that her husband wouldn't *admit* it, so they would have to beat him until he did. After several beatings, the bewildered woodcutter agreed he was a doctor and started his practice. So, like the woodcutter, I took on the mantle and started to study genital herpes infection.

It turns out that genital and oral herpes infections are quite similar. They just occur in different places. Herpes simplex virus type 2 (HSV-2) is the usual cause of genital herpes (table 1). The virus enters in the genital area and establishes its home in the sacral nerve cell body (a spinal nerve that innervates the pelvic area and leg). The triggers for recurrences of genital herpes are less well understood then those for oral herpes, however.

Before long, I was regularly seeing patients at their request. I was particularly struck by the plight of young women with genital herpes, whose major concern was infecting their newborn babies. The stealth strategy of HSV-2 is to reactivate and move silently into genital secretions. It can thus infect an infant during its passage through the birth canal. Newborn infection is particularly severe, affecting all systems, including the brain. I saw my first case of newborn infection soon after I arrived in Utah, and I will never forget it. The infection caused such severe brain damage that the infant was left in a permanent semicomatose state.

I could easily understand the fears of women with genital herpes infection. Little was known about how to prevent newborn infection, so I decided to focus my studies on women with genital herpes.

In 1980, I was recruited back to CDC to work in the Venereal Diseases Division, where I became the "herpes expert." Because CDC considered the word *venereal* to be stigmatizing, it eventually dropped its use in favor of the term *sexually transmitted diseases*.

It was the pre-AIDS era then, and the press rarely reported STD stories. But genital herpes had aroused public interest, so television and print media reporters frequently interviewed me about it. In some of the stories, I was referred to as either Dr. Herpes or Dr. Condom. The resulting stories were very sensational, with variations on the theme "Sexual revolution causes epidemic of new, incurable STD." I became leery about talking to the media. In August 1982, *Time* magazine published an issue featuring the word *herpes* in bright red on the cover, with the subtitle "Today's Scarlet Letter." The allusion, of course, was to Hawthorne's novel in which Hester Prynne is punished for adultery by having to wear a scarlet "A" embroidered on her dress. The *Time* story and others contributed to the national hysteria about herpes, and there was a demand that the government "do something about it."

Then I was invited to appear on a popular afternoon talk show, *The Phil Donahue Show*. I had never seen it, and I was reluctant to appear because of the controversy my previous media interviews had generated. The producers insisted that if I appeared I could tell the world what CDC was doing about the genital herpes "epidemic." I finally accepted when I found out that a former CDC colleague, Larry Corey, MD, a prominent herpesvirus researcher from Seattle, would also be on the show. I thought that between the two of us we might be able to reduce the hysteria and educate the public.

But the show turned out to be a nightmare. The live audience consisted of groups of people with an interest in the subject, some who believed that the "government was covering up the herpes epidemic." They were there for a fight. I had absolutely no understanding of what their issues were, and as the show progressed, it became clear that the host was more interested in controversy than in education. During a commercial break, Donahue ran up and down the aisles with his microphone, urging the audience to get involved. "Get 'em," he kept saying, referring to us, the invited guests.

I was embarrassed and shaken as the show resumed. Then Donahue said something to me about CDC's covering up the herpes epidemic, and the crowd started screaming. The general chaos continued until the show was finally over. I had not had any media training and was ill prepared to deal with a professional showman whose main interest was to entertain his national audience.

When a representative of the television program *60 Minutes* asked me for an interview, I politely declined. Despite his persistence, I absolutely refused. He eventually contacted the director of CDC and asked why CDC was "covering up" the herpes epidemic, so the director requested that I appear on the program. The CBS team filmed the episode in my office over a several-hour period and scheduled it to air six weeks later.

During that interval, my colleagues were worried about how CDC would be portrayed, given the show's tendency to make the interviewee look like the "bad guy." I was more worried about what my mother would think. My mother was a religious woman who had never even mentioned the word *sex* in our household. Although she knew that I worked at CDC, she had no idea what kind of work I was doing. My husband suggested that I tell my mother about the content of the program before it aired. He worried that she might have a heart attack if she wasn't warned in advance. But I could not bring myself to do it.

The televised episode opened with the question, "Dr. Guinan, which venereal disease would you least like to have?" Because I had never been asked that question during the interview, the response that was aired was a contrived one, a sliced-together collage of clips discussing syphilis, gonorrhea, genital herpes, and orogenital sex. I cringed.

When the program ended, my mother called from New York and said, "Congratulations, dear. Your hair looked very nice." She didn't touch the subject matter. But her reaction was positive, so I took that as approval. I never again worried about what people thought about my working in STDs. I received many letters responding to the program, including several that thanked me for having the courage to acknowledge publicly that I had a venereal disease.

My research in herpesviruses would eventually lead to my becoming part of the CDC task force investigating the emerging AIDS epidemic. The first formal report to CDC about the new disease came from Michael Gottlieb, MD, at the University of California, San Francisco; he had cared for five gay men who suffered with the new syndrome. In early 1981, the Epidemic Intelligence Service (EIS) officer in San Francisco called the office of CDC's weekly newsletter, the *MMWR*, and asked if it would publish the report. The editor told him that the report had to be reviewed and cleared by a unit at CDC with expertise in the subject matter, which presented a problem because no unit had such expertise. Because one of the infections reported in the patients was cytomegalovirus (a herpesvirus), it was sent to me for review. (In fact, early on, cytomegalovirus was suspected of causing the syndrome.)

MMWR published the report in June 1981 (4). The story was a milestone, not only because it was the first report of the new disease but also because it marked the first time the publication used the word *homosexual*. I thought the title should include the words *homosexual men*, but I was overruled. The title of the article was "*Pneumocystis carinii* Pneumonia, San Francisco." (In another herpes connection, Kaposi's sarcoma, which is an AIDS-related condition, was discovered in 1994 to be caused by a herpesvirus [now called HHV-8].)

As to what happened to the search for a cold sore treatment, others continued the research. Oral acyclovir was found to be an effective treatment for both oral and genital herpes infection, and the Food and Drug Administration approved it in 1982. It is a wonderful drug. At the first symptom of a cold sore, I start taking a daily dose. At minimum, acyclovir will reduce the size and duration of the cold sores. If I start early enough, no sore will appear. I never leave home without it.

An interesting aside is that Gertrude Elion, an American biochemist and pharmacologist who was one of the few women engaged in herpesvirus research, received the Nobel Prize for Physiology or Medicine in 1988, partly for her work on herpesviruses and the development of acyclovir.*

Reviewing my interactions with the media in those years—and how inaccurate their reports often were—is a painful experience. It illustrates that both audiences and news reporters were less informed on medical matters back then. To the average reader or viewer, a herpesvirus was a herpesvirus was a herpesvirus; the distinctions of type were meaningless.

And the medical community was also less sophisticated about messaging and communication skills. In 1984, when CDC held a press conference on AIDS, it was the agency's first press conference in seven years. CDC even eschewed press releases, preferring to publish its findings in "the staid, tradition-honored *MMWR*," where the newsworthy bits were often placed deep in the editorial notes, not in attention-grabbing leads (5).

And it was not until 1987 that CDC hired an expert—former EIS officer Bruce Dan, MD (known as Dr. Dan to his Chicago audience, where he was medical director for an ABC affiliate station)—to teach medical staff about using SOCOs (single, overriding communications objectives), keeping medical information simple, and learning to "flag" key messages (6).

---

*Gertrude Elion was also a graduate of Hunter College, majored in chemistry, and upon graduation could not find work in her field—all experiences that I shared (see chapter 2).

So I have come not to blame Dan Rather, but to thank him for pushing me into a detour that became a career. He also gave me an important early warning about the perils of scientists trying to communicate to the media on health issues. Now I can laugh when people call me Dr. Herpes.

FIVE

Healthcare Workers and Enemy Information in a War Zone, Pakistan, 1980

IN DECEMBER 1979, the Soviet Union sent Russian military forces to Afghanistan to prop up a Soviet-friendly government that was in danger of falling to rebels. This invasion was another ploy in the ongoing Cold War between the United States and the Soviet Union and their respective allies.

The United States responded immediately by suspending nuclear arms negotiations and condemning the invasion at the United Nations (UN). In March 1980, President Jimmy Carter announced that the United States would boycott the summer Olympic Games in Moscow unless the Soviets retreated. There was no retreat.

Russian forces in Afghanistan would soon number over 100,000. Soviet-led Afghan troops fought multinational insurgent groups called the Mujahideen. The fierce fighting resulted in thousands of Afghans fleeing over the borders to the neighboring countries of Iran and Pakistan. In the months after the invasion, tens of thousands of refugees were in Pakistan, camping in the area of the Khyber Pass close to the Afghan border in North-West Frontier Province (now known as Khyber Pakhtunkhwa Province). The lack of resources in this remote area and the soaring population of women and children in the refugee camps created international concern for their safety. There were reports that the Russian troops had crossed the border into Pakistan in "hot pursuit" of the Mujahideen. Pakistan President Muhammad Zia-ul-Haq was a supporter of the

Mujahideen in the fight against the Soviet Union, and Pakistan became an important US ally.

In April 1980, I was working in CDC's sexually transmitted disease (STD) unit when I received a call from my supervisor. The US State Department had requested CDC's assistance in evaluating the condition of Afghan refugees in Pakistani camps, and CDC wanted me to lead a team to accomplish this mission.

I was dumbfounded. I had no particular expertise in refugees. Moreover, I had just returned from a month's tour at the American University of Beirut, where I had been particularly unlucky. Lebanon was in the midst of an ongoing civil war between Muslim and Christian factions, and I had been caught in the middle of machine gun fire from a militia group that was invading the university hospital emergency room, where I happened to be. Fortunately, the soldiers were not shooting directly at us but above our heads. As rounds of bullets ricocheted off the high cement walls, I instinctively fell to the floor, where I found myself with a group of women (either patients or visitors), none of whom could speak English. Since I could not speak Arabic, we were unable to exchange information on what was going on. The shooting lasted about five minutes. Then the soldiers left, and everyone got up and continued what they had been doing before the interruption. I never found out which militia it was or why they were shooting, but the experience dampened my enthusiasm for traveling to another war-torn area for any reason.

And lastly, my boss did not want me to go to Pakistan. I had been out of the country enough. Now it was time to do STD work. I was preparing to attend the world conference of the UN Decade for Women in Copenhagen in July 1980, where I would represent the STD unit.

The State Department had specific criteria for the team leader. It wanted a woman physician, trained in infectious diseases, who had international experience. Why a woman? Because the refugees were primarily Muslim women; cultural mores would preclude an unrelated man from entering their encampments. Why me? Because I was the only woman physician at CDC with infectious diseases training and international experience. It was all very vague. I said I would think about it.

Hearing of my reluctance to commit, someone from high up in the CDC hierarchy called to discuss the mission. He told me it would be difficult for CDC to refuse the State Department's request. The pressure was on, and so I reluctantly agreed to go. Another woman physician from CDC, Mary Serdula, MD, would be going with me. She called to get more information, and I told her I knew next to nothing about it. I never spoke to anyone at the State Department, and the paucity of information on what the two of us were expected to do was disconcerting.

We heard nothing more for weeks. Then in late May/early June, the process began. CDC briefed Dr. Serdula and me on what we should be doing in the camps to assess the health status of the refugees. We were given various field supplies, including an instrument to measure the height and weight of children. We reviewed and modified a questionnaire that we would administer to the refugees through an interpreter.

Our first stop was Washington, DC, where we had a two-day briefing by various State Department officials, including the so-called desk officers (foreign service officers who are in-house experts on each country) for Pakistan and Afghanistan. From Washington we boarded a flight to Islamabad, the capital of Pakistan.

While being driven from the airport to our hotel, we passed by the remains of the American Embassy. Pakistani students had burned it to the ground just seven months before (on November 22, 1979). Four people at the embassy had been killed—two Americans and two Pakistanis. The embassy was relocated temporarily to the

Agency for International Development offices in another part of Islamabad. Security at the new location was extremely tight.

During the next few days, Dr. Serdula and I met with various embassy officials and reviewed the game plan. At lunch and dinner, we heard ghastly details about the burning of the embassy from workers who had escaped the building. Two weeks before the burning of that embassy, a mob had stormed the American Embassy in Iran (on November 4, 1979) and taken fifty-two American hostages, who were still being held in captivity. (They would not be released until January 1981.) There was great relief that no hostages had been taken in Islamabad. Because of the danger, we did not leave our hotel except when accompanied by someone from the embassy.

We outlined what we were supposed to do. We were to go the camps and collect information from the refugees that would identify their greatest health-related needs. Using this information, the State Department would determine what resources would be sent to Pakistan.

The embassy made all the arrangements for our travel. We would be driving about 90 miles with a caravan to Peshawar, capital of North-West Frontier Province, on a fairly reasonable but crowded road. Why so many embassy personnel were accompanying us was unclear. But given the political turmoil, I assumed it was for security reasons, and I was grateful.

Peshawar is an ancient city close to the Afghanistan border. It had been part of Afghanistan until 1957, when the British incorporated it into North-West Frontier Province. Because of its strategic location, it has been a center of trade for centuries between central and south Asia. It is the administrative and economic center for the Federally Administered Tribal Areas. Most recently, Peshawar has been in the news because of the brutal Taliban massacre of 132 schoolchildren in 2014. But Peshawar was violent, even then.

The camps we were to visit required passage through a number of these tribal areas. We stayed in Peshawar for a few days while the necessary documents were obtained for our travel through each tribal area. The leaders of each tribal area would be responsible for our safe passage through their territory, and each of them would have to approve our passage. There was apparently a limit to how many persons could be in our travel party, so several of those who traveled with us to Peshawar did not continue on to the camps.

After a breathtaking drive on a narrow road in the Hindu Kush mountain range, we arrived at the first tribal area. There we were met by tribal leaders, who welcomed us and assigned us a bodyguard with a rifle and bandoleer to protect us while we were under their jurisdiction. This process was repeated at each successive tribal area. We stayed overnight in two of these tribal areas in government rest houses.

At the second tribal area, while we were arranging our lodging, the leader of the State Department group (whom I will call Bob) told Dr. Serdula and me that several of the people traveling with us were Central Intelligence Agency (CIA) agents. As the conversation continued, it became clear that we were being used as a cover so that the CIA could gather information on what was going on at the border. We were quite shaken and bewildered by this information and asked why we hadn't been told previously. Bob said he was telling us now so that we would know. Neither of us would have agreed to go had we known the real mission of the expedition.

We had no choice but to keep going and do what we had been trained to do. Because the refugees were Pathans, a group of nomadic people who live on both sides of the Afghanistan-Pakistan border, we needed an interpreter who spoke Pushtu, their native language. One was assigned to us in Peshawar, a young man who had a name that we could not pronounce. (When we asked him for

an English translation of his name, he told us, "Slave of the Prophet.")
I told Bob while we were in Peshawar that I had specifically requested a female interpreter because a man would not be allowed
into the tents of the women. He said that he had difficulty finding
a woman and was still working on it, but we would have to use
Slave of the Prophet for the time being. So the male interpreter
accompanied us to the camp.

The site of the camp was a large barren area, where tents had
been set up for the refugees. The tents were not close to one another. It was extremely hot—well over 100 degrees Fahrenheit all
day. Dr. Serdula and I wore light cotton clothes that we had had
made for us in a local shop in Islamabad. They were wide pants and
long shirts that reached below our knees, much like the clothing
that many Muslim women wear. We also bought headscarves.

The sun made it almost unbearable to work in the heat of the
day, so we worked mainly in the early morning and in the evening.
We selected an area for the interviews and then numbered the
tents. We decided on visiting every fifth tent to interview the occu-
pants, most of whom were women and children. Finally, the female
interpreter arrived. The women welcomed us and were very cooperative in answering our questions. After the interviews, we also mea-
sured the height and weight of each child with the instrument provided to us by CDC. The measuring process was conducted outside
the tent and usually attracted a crowd of people.

After the first few days, we had questions from many women
about why we did not come to *their* tents. It was difficult to explain,
and we never really knew what the interpreter told them. The interpreter was linked to a political family that was no longer in a position
of power. She wore a beautiful white dress and showed little empathy
for the refugees, and we were sometimes concerned whether she was
accurately representing their or our words.

Dr. Serdula and I worked for almost a week, and then we were told it was time to leave. A few days before we left, a group of men in the camp asked to speak with me. The leader thanked us for coming and for being concerned about their health, but he said that they needed more help. He asked me to tell the president when I returned to the United States that they needed "guns to fight the Haj." (*Haj* means "holy war.") I told him that I would deliver his message.

We returned through the tribal areas to Peshawar, where we stayed a few days to write our report. Bob and his group went back to Islamabad. We reviewed all the data that we had collected and prepared a draft report with recommendations. Then we flew to Islamabad. Dr. Serdula went home, but I stayed a few days, working at the embassy to complete the report.

I refused to believe that the only purpose of our trip was to give the CIA access to the war zone. After all, we had accumulated reasonable information on the status of the refugees, which might be useful in making decisions on resources. I gave the full report with all the collected data to a top embassy aide and asked that he put in on the ambassador's desk. I then left for Copenhagen and the UN Decade for Women conference. I never found out whether anyone read the report. Maybe it is better not to know.

A few years ago, I ran into Dr. Serdula at a CDC meeting, and the first thing we discussed was how we had been used by the CIA. We both still felt terrible about it, almost like they had stolen part of our souls. We were supposed to be the "good guys."

The CIA again used public health workers in Pakistan in 2011. According to an editorial in *Scientific American*, titled "How the CIA's Fake Vaccination Campaign Endangers Us All," the CIA, hoping to identify Osama bin Laden's family, used a sham hepatitis B vaccination project to collect DNA from residents in Abbottabad who were living close to bin Laden's suspected hideout (1). After bin Laden's capture and death on May 2, 2011, the fake scheme came to light, and villagers along the Afghanistan-Pakistan border chased off vaccination workers, accusing them of being spies.

The misuse of public health workers had repercussions. In December 2012, nine female Pakistani workers were gunned down while administering polio vaccinations, prompting the UN to withdraw vaccination teams. A similar attack occurred in Nigeria in February 2013, when nine female vaccination workers were massacred. These attacks are presumed to be retaliation for the vaccinator ruse in the capture of bin Laden.

In January 2013, several deans of US schools of public health signed a letter to President Barack Obama stating their belief that public health programs should not be used as cover for covert operations and urging the president to assure the public that this type of practice would not be repeated (2). The president did not respond.

While working on AIDS in Africa, I encountered widespread belief that the CIA had deliberately put the AIDS virus into vaccines in order to kill Africans. In India during the smallpox eradication program, women in some villages would run away when they saw us coming because they believed vaccination was a family planning plot to sterilize them. I was certain then, and still am, that these suspicions were totally unfounded. I mention these events only because they illustrate how suspicions about the West and its medicine are rife in many countries, especially underdeveloped ones. We only lend credence to such fears when public health workers are used for political purposes.

SIX

An AIDS Needlestick at a Rundown Hotel in San Francisco, 1982

THE HOTEL was close to Skid Row, in the Tenderloin District of San Francisco, and it reflected the seediness of the area. The fact that the clothes washer and dryer for hotel guests were located in the lobby, one on either side of the registration desk, gives you some idea.

I had chosen the hotel because I could get a room with a refrigerator within the federal government rate (about $45 per day in 1982), and because it was directly across the street from the post office. One pleasant feature was a back courtyard with tables and chairs, where one could enjoy the beautiful autumn weather. My room was on the second floor, with a deck overlooking the courtyard, and I could walk around it between interviews.

Several months after CDC reported the first cases of what eventually would be called AIDS (1), I conducted my part of the first case-control study of the new disease in this hotel. I was one of the thirty people in CDC's Kaposi's Sarcoma and Opportunistic Infections (KSOI) Task Force, which led the study. Four cities were included in the study: Atlanta, Los Angeles, New York, and San Francisco.

The protocol was the same in each city. We were to interview a male homosexual patient diagnosed with Kaposi's sarcoma or *Pneumocystis* pneumonia, four healthy homosexual controls, and one heterosexual control. All of the controls were matched by city of residence, gender, race, and age to the patient with Kaposi's sarcoma or

Pneumocystis pneumonia. Therefore, for each case-control unit, there were six interviews, each conducted by the same person.

From tryouts with the form, we expected each interview to last from one to two hours and the collection of specimens at least another half hour. I calculated that the maximum number of interviews I could do in any one day was four—if everything went smoothly. I interviewed each study participant using the approved form.

If written permission were given, I obtained various specimens, including blood, urine, and oral and rectal swabs. For processing, the specimens had to arrive at CDC's laboratories within twenty-four hours, so I sent them by the post office's overnight mail. The most fragile—and perhaps most important—specimen was blood, particularly the lymphocytes, the cells that seemed to be destroyed by whatever was causing the disease.

The study was an extensive undertaking. We worked in concert with the established local public health network of city, county, and state health department personnel, who handled most of the logistics. The local health departments first recruited the patients for the study and then found age-matched control volunteers from clinics and private practitioners.

My contact in San Francisco was a public health advisor named Sal. Before I arrived from Atlanta, he had been recruiting the patients and controls. After I registered at the hotel, Sal arrived with large cartons of supplies that CDC had sent in advance to the health department. These included needles, syringes, blood tubes, containers for urine specimens, culture tubes with special media that would preserve the culture specimen for a day or so, alcohol swabs, tourniquets, bandages, gauze swabs, Styrofoam mailing containers, tape, interview forms, and odds and ends. Sal also brought a cooler with dry ice.

I set up shop in the kitchenette of my hotel room, which had a counter with stools. I placed all the supplies for taking specimens on one end of the counter near the wall. At the other end of the counter was a stool, on which the study participants would sit, placing their arms on the counter so I could draw blood.

Depending on the time of day, specimens were either refrigerated or packed in dry ice in the Styrofoam mailing containers and taken to the post office, whose posted closing was 5:00 p.m. (Actually, the doors closed at 4:45 p.m.) I walked (sometimes ran) to the post office with the specimens before closing. At first, I tried to send the specimens immediately following each interview, but I found that the lines in the post office were often so long that I would be late for my next interview. Specimens obtained later in the day would be refrigerated until morning, then packaged up and brought to the post office when it opened at 8:00 a.m.

Sal set up just two interviews the first day, with plenty of time in between to get everything done. After that, the goal was to conduct three or four interviews per day. At that rate, working seven days a week, I should be able to finish my part in two weeks (six case-control units, or thirty interviews). Each day was a little bit easier, but I usually worked from 8:00 a.m. to 10:00 p.m., leaving little time for anything else.

The young men at the hotel registration desk knew that I was from CDC and working on the "new disease." I explained to them that participants in the study would be coming to the registration desk, and I asked the clerk to call my room to see if I was ready. Often a participant would come early and bring friends. They were directed to the courtyard to wait, where they often met other participants and struck up conversations.

I always marveled at these young men who volunteered for the study. Each took a day of his life to come to the hotel to be interviewed by a federal government employee, who was asking about every aspect of his life, including highly sensitive questions on sexual behavior and drug use. Afterward, the volunteer donated the requested specimens. Although the participants were guaranteed confidentiality, the process was still a considerable invasion of privacy.

Invariably, each participant expressed his reason for participating as "wanting to help." The San Francisco gay population was well informed concerning the new disease. One openly gay newspaper columnist, Randy Shilts, dedicated his columns to the unfolding story of the disease. Many of the San Francisco study participants had called Randy to let him know that they were part of the study and that I would be interviewing them. He also interviewed those who contacted him and found out not only what questions I had asked but also what they had answered. One of the men I interviewed told me he would be interviewed by Randy the next day, which was concerning because public revelations about questions in a study before it is completed could compromise the answers of future participants. But Randy was careful not to reveal information he obtained until well after the study was completed and published. He eventually wrote the book *And the Band Played On* (2); the book and subsequent movie covered this study and my work there.* I

*The experience of having an event in my life portrayed in a movie was disconcerting. HBO previewed the film for CDC personnel, but I was out of town and did not see it. Upon my return, many colleagues tried to break it to me gently that I was not portrayed well. "Brace yourself" was a common comment, followed by "It isn't at all like you." When I finally did see it, I saw my character as a nice, soft-spoken woman who made a cake for a colleague. The scriptwriter simply did not know how to portray a woman scientist. In the film, Richard Gere plays a patient who kisses me on the cheek.

Every year on World AIDS Day (December 1), different memorial events are staged around the country. Sometimes the movie *And the Band Played On* is shown, accompanied by a panel of real-life characters depicted in the movie. Afterward, there are often question-and-answer sessions between panel members and attendees. I have been a panel member for several of these events—in Atlanta, Las Vegas, and Reno. People line up to talk to me. They tell me personal stories or ask questions. The question I am most commonly asked is, "Did you really kiss Richard Gere?" I was so startled when I was first asked this question that I didn't know how to respond. Now I am prepared. I say, "No, I didn't kiss Richard Gere. He kissed me." So much for my scientific expertise!

found it very difficult to read in his book the claims of my interviewing certain persons and their detailed responses—information
I would never have disclosed. In short, CDC kept the confidentiality, but Randy, who was a reporter, not a scientist, did not promise
confidentiality.

During the second week of the study, one man cancelled his
interview, giving me time to do my laundry and get some exercise.
It was great to have a break. It was the first time I had had for exercise since coming to San Francisco. (Needless to say, the hotel did
not have an exercise facility.) I put on my running clothes, put most
of the rest of my clothes into the washer in the lobby, and went out
for a run. When I returned, the washer was empty. Hoping against
hope, I checked the dryer. Nothing. The wet clothes had disap-
peared, never to be found, despite efforts by hotel personnel throughout my stay. I conducted the next interview in my running clothes—
a t-shirt and shorts—with apologies.

One evening, after interviewing a very tall patient who was built
like a football player, I stood in front of him, drawing his blood as
he sat on the stool. While the needle was in his vein and the blood
running into the tube, he fainted and fell forward on top of me. As
we both fell to the floor, I tried to open the tourniquet to stop the
pressure on the vein but I couldn't. I pulled the syringe and needle
out. When we hit the floor, my right arm with the syringe hit first
and pushed the needle into the palm of my left hand. Because the
tourniquet was still in place, blood was running down the patient's
shirt. I finally undid the tourniquet, but not before both the patient
and I were covered with blood. I checked him, and his breathing
and pulse were fine.

I washed the needlestick wound in my palm with alcohol and
tried to squeeze out any of the patient's blood that might be inside.
But I was preoccupied with other things. I was in a sleazy hotel,
wearing a bloody blouse, with an unconscious man on the floor

covered with blood, and syringes and needles on the counter. I hoped the patient would come to quickly so I wouldn't have to call for help. The situation would be very difficult to explain.

Fortunately, he awakened. Embarrassed and apologetic, he explained that he usually fainted at the site of blood and was sorry that he had not warned me. I apologized about his shirt.

Because I had not yet collected the needed blood specimens, I asked if I could draw blood from the other arm while he was still lying on the floor. He agreed. Afterward he got up and cleaned himself off, sat for a while, and then left. I was amazed at his cooperation.

I did not think too much about the needlestick then. We knew neither the cause of the disease nor its mode of spread at that point. Our working hypothesis was that either an infectious agent or an environmental agent such as a drug or drug combination was causing the observed paucity of certain blood lymphocytes that resulted in immunosuppression in patients. I completed my interviews during the third week and went home, carrying the hard copy of all the data on my lap on the airplane. The results of this study were published in 1983 (3).

In 1984, the virus that causes AIDS was identified and eventually named the human immunodeficiency virus (HIV). A blood test was being developed to identify patients who were infected.

On November 29, 1984, approximately two years after the needlestick, I found a spot on my left arm that looked very much like a lesion of Kaposi's sarcoma—an AIDS diagnosis. It was purple, raised above the skin, and painless to the touch. By this time, it was known that a stick from a needle that was used in a person with AIDS could transmit the virus.

I was frightened but tried to keep calm. I had given birth to my son the previous year, and I knew that the risk of transmission of HIV from an infected mother to her newborn was 30 percent. My son was perfectly healthy. If I were infected, there was also a great risk that I had infected my husband. But he too was healthy. Despite these two auspicious signs, the incubation period from time of infection with the virus to the development of signs and symptoms of AIDS, though not yet well delineated, was thought to average two to ten years. It was still quite possible that I had contracted the disease.

My husband was on a field trip in Mexico, and I could not contact him. (This was well before the availability of cell phones or e-mail.) I went to work that day and showed the lesion to a colleague (the late Sam Thompson, MD). He worked at CDC and at the infectious diseases unit at Emory University School of Medicine, and he had taken care of many AIDS patients. When he looked at the lesion, I saw his expression change. He touched it and asked if it hurt. I said no.

"You have to get that biopsied immediately," he said, confirming my fear. I wanted another opinion and drove to another facility at CDC, where Harold Jaffe, MD, worked. He also had been part of the KSOI Task Force. He was busy, and his secretary did not want to interrupt him. I insisted, saying it was urgent. He came out of his office, somewhat annoyed. I showed him my arm. He touched the lesion and looked at me.

"Do you remember the needlestick?" I asked.

"You need to have that biopsied immediately," he answered.

"Harold, do you think it's possible?" I asked.

"Yes," he said. "It is possible."

I went back to my office and called a dermatologist friend to get an appointment. He was not in town, and his receptionist said he would not be back until the next week. I made an appointment for the following Tuesday, December 4. Five days later.

In the meantime, one of CDC's top administrators came to my office. Obviously, he had been notified. As he was speaking to me, my secretary came into the office. "I heard that you have AIDS," she said. She was very upset and said she was sorry, but she could no longer work for me because she had three children and couldn't take the risk. She took her purse and left.

The administrator advised me to get a biopsy as soon as possible. I called other dermatologists but could not get an earlier appointment. It turned out that the annual meeting of the American College of Dermatology was being held in Washington, DC, the following weekend, and most of the dermatologists in Atlanta were either there or en route. It was unlikely I would have a biopsy before Tuesday.

I went home. Physically, I felt fine. If I had the infection, shouldn't I have other symptoms? Or was I deluding myself?

On Friday, a number of colleagues visited my office and expressed their concern. The word had spread. I explained that I would have to wait for the biopsy.

Later that day, Jim Curran, MD, the director of the CDC AIDS Program, called me. He expressed his concern and offered me the possibility of having my blood tested anonymously for HIV at CDC's laboratories. Although the test was not yet approved by the Food and Drug Administration and not available commercially, CDC was using it. I thought about this. I asked how it would be possible to keep the specimen anonymous. He said, "We will put a number on it." I said, "Well, what number are you going to put, number 1?" Someone in the lab would know it was my blood being tested no matter what the number was. I told him no, thank you. I was not ready. I said I would wait for the biopsy.

I spent the weekend worrying. By Sunday, the lesion appeared to be smaller. Or was that my imagination? But on Monday it was barely detectable. By Tuesday, it was gone. I knew then that I did not have Kaposi's sarcoma because those lesions do not go away. I shook off the mantle of fear I had been carrying and celebrated by canceling the dermatology appointment. What a relief.

However, I neglected to tell my colleagues, who later in the week asked about the results of the biopsy. I showed them my arm. No sign of the lesion. We speculated that the lesion might have been caused by a spider bite.

Everything turned out well, although my secretary found another job and did not return to CDC. It took me a year to get up the courage to be tested for HIV. The test result was negative.

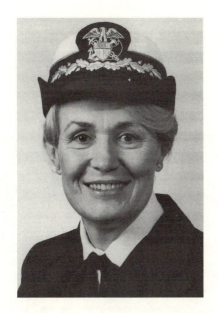

The author in captain's uniform as a Commission Corps officer of the US Public Health Service, 1984. David J. Sencer CDC Museum

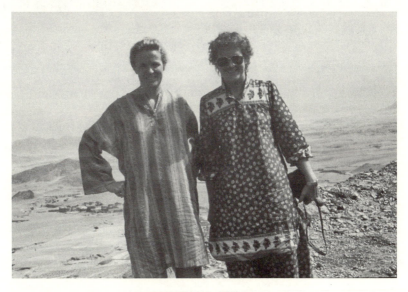

Drs. Mary Guinan (*left*) and Mary Serdula (*right*) in the North-West Frontier Province of Pakistan, 1980. Dr. Serdula's collection

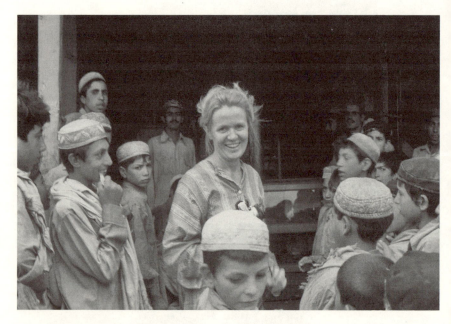

Dr. Guinan, in traditional dress, in an Afghan refugee
camp in Pakistan, 1980. Dr. Serdula's collection

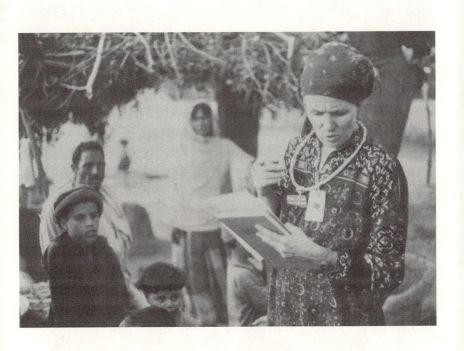

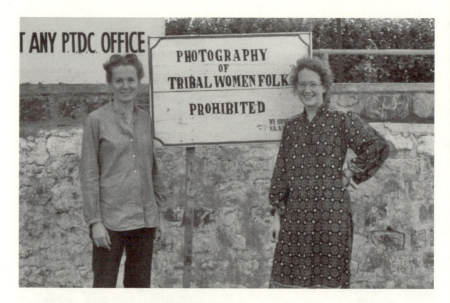

Drs. Mary Guinan (*left*) and Mary Serdula (*right*) visiting
Pakistani refugee camps, 1980. Dr. Serdula's collection

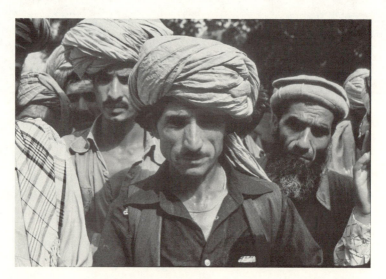

Mujahideen in an Afghan refugee camp, asking for weapons to fight
the Haj, 1980. Dr. Serdula's collection

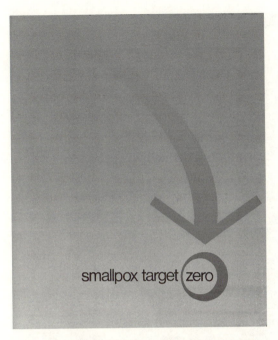

WHO Smallpox Zero poster published in 1972. This poster coincided with the launching of what was termed the "final phase," which at that time was optimistically expected to result in eradication by the summer of 1974. Copyright WHO, all rights reserved

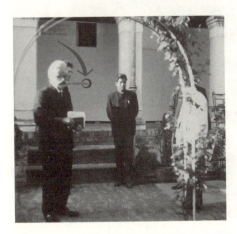

Shafi Muhammad (*middle*), Dr. Guinan's invaluable paramedical assistant in Uttar Pradash (UP), stands in front of the UP smallpox office; the Smallpox Zero poster is just visible in background, 1975. Author's collection

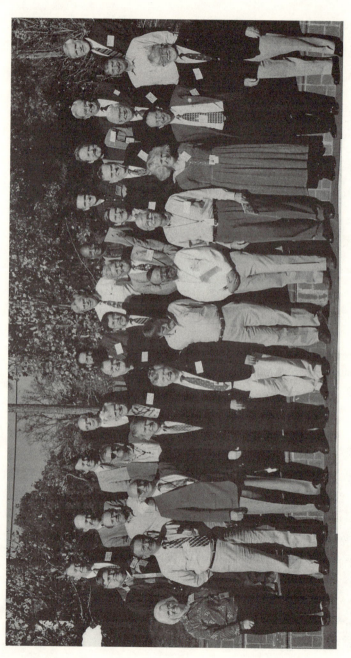

Twentieth-anniversary celebration of the eradication of smallpox by the "smallpox warriors," as then–Surgeon General David Satcher, MD, PhD, called them, CDC, 1997. Author is third from right, bottom row. *Second from right,* Dr. Walt Orenstein. *Top right,* Dr. Bill Foege, director of the Indian smallpox eradication effort in which the author participated. David J. Sencer CDC Museum

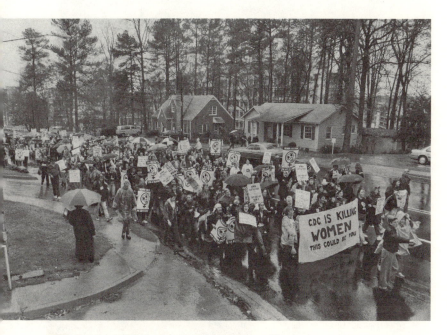

ACT UP protesters at CDC, December 3, 1990. *Atlanta Journal Constitution*; available from Georgia State University / University Library Special Collections and Archives, digital collection

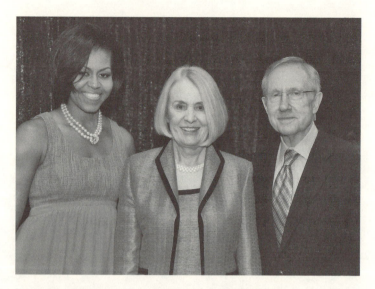

Dr. Guinan spoke on women's health at the Women's Summit in Reno, Nevada, in 2012, sponsored by Senator Harry Reid. First Lady Michelle Obama was the keynote speaker. Author's collection

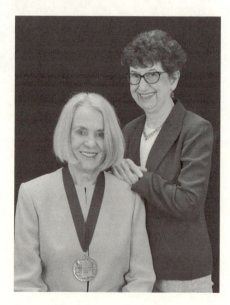

Dr. Janet Osuch of the American Medical Women's Association *(right)* awards Dr. Guinan the 2014 Elizabeth Blackwell Medal. This award is granted annually to the woman physician "who has made the most outstanding contributions to the cause of women in the field of medicine." Author's collection

SEVEN

ACT UP Acts Up at CDC over the Definition of AIDS for Women

THE AIDS Coalition to Unleash Power, or ACT UP, was formed by the gay community in New York City in 1987 after prodding from Larry Kramer, a prominent gay writer and political activist. Kramer challenged gays to fight the perceived indifference of the public to the devastation of their communities from AIDS.

ACT UP was a "direct action" group. Its members wanted to be heard, and their demonstrations at government and corporate entities were loud and boisterous (though nonviolent). ACT UP protests caused sufficient chaos from its "in-your-face," confrontational approach that many people were arrested. In fact, one of the group's main objectives *was* to get protesters arrested: the larger the number, the more likely the media attention. ACT UP was extremely effective in getting its message across. The group's demonstrations at the Food and Drug Administration, the National Institutes of Health, and pharmaceutical companies often resulted in successful negotiations for ACT UP issues.

A group of ACT UP members focused on women's issues concerning human immunodeficiency virus (HIV) and AIDS. Because lesbians were actually at a lower risk for HIV than heterosexual women, ACT UP women saw their mission as acting on behalf of all women. (Many black women with HIV/AIDS did not share this view. I heard them angrily denounce ACT UP at meetings on the grounds that the group did not speak for them.) ACT UP's main goal was to change the case definition of AIDS.

A case definition is a set of uniform criteria used to define a disease for public health monitoring purposes. (It is specifically *not* intended to be used by healthcare providers for individual patients' healthcare needs.) CDC uses case definitions to classify and count cases consistently across reporting jurisdictions. Only the state has the authority to require reporting of diseases from healthcare providers, laboratories, or public health agencies. CDC requests that states report certain diseases of public health concern, and then, in cooperation with state and local health authorities, develops the case definition. Having a clear, standardized case definition is a fundamental principle of both public health surveillance and epidemiologic investigations.

I had first encountered the ACT UP women at the 1987 International AIDS Conference in Washington, DC, where I was presenting the first CDC study on women with AIDS in the United States, which included over 1,800 women (1). After my presentation, a group of ACT UP women approached me and asked whether I would support changing the AIDS case definition to include a disease or condition that was specific to women. I pointed out that my study indicated that there was *not* a woman-specific disease that would identify women with AIDS.

They were unhappy with my response. Their position was that women were dying of AIDS but were not being counted because CDC did not count women's diseases and conditions. How this led to the claim that CDC was "killing women" was not clear. I agreed that women with AIDS were probably undercounted, but I discussed how the new HIV test would enable the identification of HIV-infected women even before they had AIDS. By this time, the scientific evidence showed that AIDS indicator diseases were actually late stages of HIV infection. CDC was then preparing a new case definition for AIDS, which would include having an HIV-positive test. I told the ACT UP women that as HIV-infected women began to be followed throughout the course of their disease, a female-specific disease or condition might be recognized. They became angry and started shouting that instead of being an advocate for women with HIV/AIDS, I was complicit with CDC in "killing women," and then they left.

I assumed that these things were said in the heat of the moment and that the issue would eventually be resolved with the new case definition. But it turned out that including a female-specific condition remained a lingering, festering issue for ACT UP. In the early investigations of AIDS, when the cause was unknown, we used the following case definition: "Kaposi's Sarcoma (KS), *Pneumocystis carinii* pneumonia (PCP) or other opportunistic infections (OI) in a patient not previously known to be immuno-suppressed." In September 1987, CDC announced a revised case definition of AIDS that did not include a woman-specific disease but did include a positive HIV test.

In January 1988, *Cosmopolitan* magazine published an article titled "Reassuring News about AIDS: A Doctor Tells Why You May Not Be at Risk" (2). Written by a psychiatrist, it essentially told women that so long as their "genitals were healthy," it was okay to have unprotected sex even if their partner were HIV positive. It was outrageous.

The story reflected a widespread belief that women could *not* get HIV/AIDS through penile-vaginal intercourse. Even among physicians and scientists there was a group that persisted in denying that women were susceptible (unless they did the "unthinkable," such as having sex in something other than the missionary position). At the same AIDS scientific meeting where I presented the study on 1,800 women with AIDS, mentioned above, a scientist from the National Institutes of Health presented a poster showing electron microscopic images of the vaginal wall that purportedly demonstrated why it protected women from HIV infection. The undercurrent of the belief was that a "good girl" could not get HIV infection. And if she did, it was because she was doing something like injecting drugs or having anal intercourse.*

In response to the *Cosmopolitan* article, the ACT UP women took action. One of the group members called me, and we discussed the article. I agreed that it was irresponsible and could do considerable harm. In fact, I had already contacted the magazine and offered to write an article on the real risk of HIV for women. *Cosmopolitan* was not interested. Nor would it publish a letter to the editor pointing out the inaccuracies in the article.

I learned that ACT UP had an appointment to meet with the author, Dr. Robert E. Gould, in New York City. They asked if I could attend. I declined, fearing the possibility of arrest if the usual group chaos occurred. Apparently, the subsequent meeting was tense, and the physician stood his ground and refused to retract his statements. The women were so angry that they were determined to "take *Cosmo* down." I shared their anger.

ACT UP planned a protest at the magazine's editorial offices. Over a hundred activists protested in front of the Hearst Tower in Manhattan. The protest was widely covered by the media and spurred a number of talk shows, including Phil Donahue's, to feature topics on HIV in women. The physician interview, the protest at *Cosmopolitan,* and the talk shows were videotaped by ACT UP women and made into the documentary film *Doctors, Liars and Women: AIDS Activists Say NO to Cosmo.* I was so pleased when I saw a news clip of the protest with signs proclaiming, "Yes, the

---

*I salute the courage of Mary Fisher, an HIV-infected, wealthy white woman who spoke at the Republican Convention in 1992, demonstrating that "nice" women can get AIDS. She is an international hero and continues to advocate for the prevention and treatment of HIV infection in women.

Cosmo Girl Can Get AIDS." Eventually, *Cosmopolitan* printed a half-hearted correction.

So I had interacted a bit with the ACT UP women. But CDC itself had yet to be targeted by the group. Then, in January 1990—a couple of years after the *Cosmo* incident—ACT UP officially set its sights on CDC. On the first day, January 8, hundreds of activists from around the country came to the state capitol in Atlanta to protest Georgia's sodomy law. The following day, the group protested in front of the CDC main building on Clifton Road.

My office was in that building, and I could see the line of chanting marchers with placards that read "CDC is killing women." The placards appeared to be handmade, and many had graphic portrayals of female genitalia. Several of the group tried to break into the building but were rebuffed by police in riot gear, including helmets and batons, who were lined up in front of the building. It was chaotic. A few protesters managed to hoist a lavender flag up the flagpole in front of CDC. In the end, close to fifty people were arrested.

Local media coverage was surprisingly sparse. Of course, the graphic placards didn't help. But I also don't think that the media understood the protesters' concerns. How exactly was CDC killing women? What was this protest about? During ACT UP protests at the National Institutes of Health and the Food and Drug Administration, the messages had been clearer: get more AIDS drugs, improve clinical trials, let HIV patients participate in experimental drug trials, fund more AIDS research. By contrast, the women from ACT UP who led the CDC protest wanted a change in the case definition of AIDS with regard to women. This was a concept not easily understood by the media or the public (nor, I suspect, by most of the protesters).

In the months following this first ACT UP demonstration, CDC met with ACT UP protesters to see if they could come to some agreement on their case definition demands. I was not involved until

I was invited to the last of these meetings. Negotiations had not gone well, and apparently the leaders asked to meet with CDC women scientists. Ruth Berkelman, MD, the deputy director of the Center for Infectious Diseases, and I were the two scientists who met with two ACT UP leaders.

It was tense right from the beginning, with ACT UP demanding that yeast vaginitis be included as an indicator disease in the AIDS case definition. We were shocked. We discussed how common yeast vaginitis is in US women without HIV infection. In fact, it is estimated that 75 percent of women in the United States will have at least one yeast vaginal infection in their lifetime. Considering the climate at the time, the inclusion of vaginal yeast infection as an AIDS indicator disease would have caused widespread panic among women. But all our reasoning fell on deaf ears. The ACT UP members abruptly left the meeting with some vague warnings.

I did not know it at the time, but CDC's refusal to budge on this case definition would precipitate the second ACT UP protest at CDC in December 1990. And this time, I would be one of the targets.

I had no further contact with the group. I changed jobs within CDC that year and moved from administration back to the HIV/AIDS unit, which was located in an office park several miles from CDC headquarters. The second ACT UP protest began at the main facility, but somehow the group discovered that my office was not there but at the office park. The protest moved to the office park, but the police were unaware of this move. The office park had no security.

When the protesters arrived, someone had the good sense to lock the glass entry door to our building, which was next to my office. We called the police. There was chaos outside; lots of people were chanting. I could not see the messages on the placards, and I was still unaware that I was a target. The police had not yet arrived, but we were locked in and felt pretty safe.

Then the unexpected occurred. The mailman came. He had a key to the building, and he opened the door. The protesters burst in. They ran all over the place, including into people's offices. I heard them ask, "Where is Mary Guinan?" My assistant whispered, "They are calling your name!" She was terrified. I took the sign with my name on it off my office door and told her to go inside and lock the door. I sat down at her desk. Fortunately, no one recognized me.

They started chanting, "Mary Guinan, you can't hide. We accuse you of gynecide." (*Gynecide* means "killing women.") The chants kept up. Fifty or so protestors were roaming through the building looking for fax machines, one of which was next to my assistant's desk. I caught a glimpse of what they were trying to send: a message to all news and media outlets, stating that CDC had relented and that vaginal yeast infection would be now part of the AIDS case definition. But they were having difficulty getting an outside line, which required a certain code. They kept pressing 9, which was the incorrect button, so the faxes did not go through.

I wondered what was keeping the police. They finally arrived, and so did the media. The police were all wearing yellow rubber gloves. (The fear of contracting AIDS had prompted the use of rubber gloves when handling AIDS protesters.) The protesters started chanting, "Your gloves don't match your shoes; they'll see it on the news." Finally, the police entered the building. The protesters lay down on the floor all over the building and would not move. They were carried out one by one by the police. The protesters kept up the chant about the gloves, alternating it with the Guinan-gynecide chant (3).

I never saw the video footage of the protests because there was minimal television coverage of the event. There was little attention paid by the print media as well, likely because they did not understand the issues surrounding a case definition. The protesters did not achieve their objective of notifying the national media that CDC had changed the AIDS case definition to include yeast vaginitis, but only because they could not get the fax machines to work. I often wonder what would have happened if they had pressed the right button to get an outside line.

The invasion of our offices seriously traumatized our employees. The employee-assistance workers set up a series of counseling sessions for all those affected. And CDC improved security in all its facilities.

For a long time after this incident, I received anonymous postcards featuring a target with my face in the middle. This was well before the Internet, but organizations had some way of communicating with people all over the nation. Subsequently, every time I gave a talk at a medical meeting, a plant would be in the audience, and it was always a woman. No matter what the subject of my lecture, someone would get up in the audience and shout, "Stop killing women!" This lasted for several years, until I left CDC.

The case definition of AIDS has changed several times. Most recently, it is defined as the late stage of HIV infection.

EIGHT

The HIV-Infected Preacher's Wife

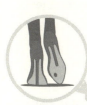

I FIRST met her when she was a patient at the infectious diseases clinic at the county health department in Georgia. *Infectious diseases* was the new name given for what used to be called sexually transmitted diseases (STDs), and before that venereal diseases (VDs). Can you imagine the courage of the patients who visited such clinics before the name change, sitting in large, open waiting rooms for hours with no privacy, subjected to the scrutiny of all who passed by? Infectious diseases was hopefully a less humiliating name.

The name change was prompted by the emergence of the AIDS epidemic in the early 1980s and the fear of people with human immunodeficiency virus (HIV) infection. One cannot exaggerate the fear and hysteria throughout the country during the 1980s concerning those infected. During this time, Ryan White, a child with hemophilia who was infected with HIV from contaminated blood products, was expelled from a middle school in Indianapolis because of his infection. Parents and teachers strongly supported keeping Ryan out of the school. In Florida, the parents of three brothers with hemophilia who were HIV positive filed a federal lawsuit against the county school board to allow their children to attend public school despite their diagnoses. Although the parents won the lawsuit in 1987, their home was burned to the ground by vigilantes, and they moved away.

If it were widely known that HIV-infected patients visited the county health department, people would likely keep away. Indeed, the coordinator of the Alcoholics Anonymous meetings at the department reported that attendance had dropped because of rumors that AIDS patients might be in the STD clinic. So the clinic changed its name.

I saw Lir* for the first time in 1986. I was the only woman physician at the clinic, and the nurses steered the female patients to me. Lir had driven over 120 miles from a small town in another state. This is her story.

She had grown up in the small town, the only child of a single mother. When Lir was in high school, her mother developed breast cancer. The family belonged to a church, and while the mother was dying, the preacher and the congregation attended to her. When her mother died, Lir was courted by the preacher, who was twenty years her senior. She eventually married him around 1980 and had two children, a boy and a girl.

Sometime later, it was revealed that the preacher was sexually molesting both of their children. The preacher pled guilty to this offense and went to the state prison. Lir was determined to keep him there for the rest of his life.

In 1985, a test for HIV became available, and soon many states began testing prisoners. One day, Lir received a call from the state prison. Her former husband had tested positive for HIV. Both she and the children must be tested. Fortunately, the children tested negative. Lir, however, was positive.

---

*Lir was not her real name. Her overriding concern to protect her children reminded me of the plight of the children in an old Irish legend, "The Children of Lir." In that legend, the children became swans. I do not know what happened to Lir's children.

Lir had not yet reached her thirtieth birthday. She was tall and thin, with beautiful eyes, pale skin, and long, straight brown hair, which she wore behind her back with a clip. When she walked, her back was so straight that it seemed like a steel rod was holding it in place. Lir worked as a waitress in a restaurant in the small town and was the sole support of herself and her children. She told me that if anyone found out she was HIV positive she would lose her job, and she believed that the children would be driven out of the elementary school. That is why she drove to Georgia, where she knew no one, for her healthcare.

On that first visit, she had no symptoms or signs of AIDS, but she knew it was just a matter of time. No effective treatments for HIV were yet available. Over the several years I saw her, she was preoccupied with what would happen to her children when she died. She had no close family, and no one except her healthcare providers knew of the HIV infection.

What kept her going was her effort to keep her former husband in prison. He was coming up for parole, and she asked the social workers at the clinic to help her write testimony against him. She had to be very careful, however. On the one hand, she wanted the parole board to know that he had infected her. On the other hand, she was terrified that such testimony would become public. So in the end she decided not to reveal that he had infected her with HIV. Even without this knowledge, her testimony convinced the parole board to deny him parole in 1989, and he would not be eligible for parole for five more years. When that time came, she vowed, she would be ready to testify again.

In the early nineties, I saw her for the last time. Her infection was stable, but treatment was still not available. She told me she could not afford to drive to Georgia anymore. Gas prices were too high, and it was difficult to get the time off work.

I asked if I could do anything to help her. She shook her head, tears rolling down her cheeks. She left before the traffic got too bad.

In 1995, a combination of antiviral medications was found to be an effective treatment for HIV. Clinic personnel contacted HIV-infected patients who were eligible for the treatment. Lir was on the list, but her phone had been disconnected. She was not listed in the telephone directory of her town. We were unable to find her.

NINE

Few Safe Places

THE NEW-YORK Historical Society's exhibition *AIDS in New York: The First Five Years* opened in 2013, thirty-two years after the first reported cases of AIDS. In his review of that event (1), writer and historian Hugh Ryan described the exhibition as minimizing the suffering of gay men, especially by soft-peddling the widespread homophobia of the time. I have not seen the exhibit, but Ryan's words brought back many memories of gay men whose suffering with AIDS was compounded by an unrelenting and vicious homophobia that seemed to sweep the country in the eighties and nineties.

Before AIDS was recognized in 1981, I worked one day a week in a local health department's sexually transmitted diseases clinic, which served many gay clients. As a member of a CDC task force, I interviewed gay men in Atlanta, New York, and San Francisco for various studies. And I worked in a clinic that treated patients with human immunodeficiency virus (HIV) and AIDS. So I knew many gay men professionally and heard their stories.

THE CHURCHGOERS

In the late 1970s, I was asked to speak about hepatitis B at a Catholic church in Atlanta, where a gay and lesbian organization met monthly. (Hepatitis B can be a chronic infection that can lead to cirrhosis and cancer of the liver.) This infection was such a problem for gay men that efficacy trials of the hepatitis B vaccine were conducted exclusively among volunteers in this group.) The church was lovely. It was located in the heart of Atlanta and surrounded by gardens of flowers in full bloom.

I was nervous before the talk, as I had never spoken at a church before. I arrived early and realized that a religious service, the Catholic Mass, was in progress. So I slipped in the back, sat down in a pew, and observed. I saw about thirty or forty men and women take Communion. At the end of the service, each person walked to the altar and embraced the priest.

My presentation was in the church basement, and I was impressed both by the group's leader, a well-informed man, and by the ensuing lively discussion on changing risky sexual behaviors. I subsequently became friendly with several of the participants, who lived in my neighborhood and whom I would see occasionally at the supermarket.

Within a decade, AIDS had arrived. One day I met one of the church-group members at the grocery store. I did not recognize him at first, because he had a large hat covering most of his forehead. Then I saw the marks on his face: multiple purple lesions indicating Kaposi's sarcoma, an AIDS diagnosis. He told me he had been evicted from his house and was living with someone he barely knew, who also had AIDS. "It is like having leprosy," he said. "Even the church rejects us." Indeed, the church would no longer permit the gay and lesbian group to meet there. This man had lost his job because of his appearance and was afraid he would become homeless. His family had disowned him.

His story was not unique. There were hundreds of men disowned by families and rejected from their places of worship. The homophobia was so open and hostile in cities across the country that there were few safe places for gay men in those years. Below are a few of their stories.

MARIO

Mario was a Hispanic laboratory technician in his late twenties who lived in San Francisco. He volunteered as a control for the first national case-control study of AIDS patients. When I took his medical history, he told me he had been gang-raped the previous year and suffered a torn rectum. Multiple complications required him to be hospitalized for more than a month. He said it was not uncommon in San Francisco for Hispanic gangs to hang around outside gay bars and attack clients, especially other Hispanic men, who were deemed "a disgrace to their community."

MOSES

Moses was an HIV-positive black teenager who lived with his parents and attended a community college in Atlanta. His father was a police officer who had told Moses that he would kill him if he ever found out his son was gay. His mother discovered that Moses was cross-dressing when she found a dress and high heels hidden in his closet. She feared for his life. Moses was desperate to find another place to live, but he could not find a job.

Moses regularly came to the county health clinic with various complaints. He did not have any connection with the gay community, and he did not want it. His sexual orientation was a deep, dark secret. He did not have a car and did not want anyone to know that he was going to the clinic. To reach it from his home, he took two buses. Sometimes he missed his clinic appointment because he didn't have bus fare. He dropped out of school and eventually killed himself with one of his father's guns.

CLAY

Clay was another clinic patient, in his early thirties. He was in terrible pain. He had AIDS wasting syndrome, a condition that includes weight loss, emaciation, and uncontrollable diarrhea. He also had many very painful oral ulcers that kept him from eating. It was difficult for him to swallow pills, and because his muscles were severely atrophied, injecting pain medications was difficult.

He was too weak to walk, so a friend brought him to the clinic in a wheelchair.

In his last days, Clay begged me to give him enough medication to see him through his final days. We had tried a morphine drip, but the morphine caused nausea and vomiting. This was before pain medicine skin patches were available, which would have limited such side effects. He had to wear adult diapers, and the persistent diarrhea caused severe chafing of his genital area. The only medication that seemed to give him relief was Valium. If the pills were crushed and mixed with warm water, he was able to sip the solution through a straw, allowing him to relax enough to get some sleep, but nothing really worked very well.

Clay's family refused to see him. His partner, the man whom he believed had infected him, left him. It was understandable that Clay welcomed death.

It's true that many good people came together to help relieve the suffering of gay men during those times. But what could they do to relieve the invisible but real wounds caused by blatant and unforgiving hatred? Years after their sons died of AIDS, mothers have told me how they will never forgive themselves for abandoning their children during the time of their greatest need.

I am thankful that I have lived to see the great advances for human rights in our country for gays and lesbians. Did AIDS play a role in these advances? I believe it did. AIDS galvanized the gay community to organize a movement that I equate with the black civil rights marches in the American South. These brave persons exposed the horrors and suffering of those discriminated against for not being heterosexual.

TEN

Expert Witness for John Doe, the Pharmacist, 1991

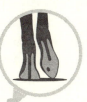

I NEVER met the hero of this story, and I do not know his real name. Nevertheless, I was an expert witness for his defense.

"John Doe" filed a complaint with the New York State Division of Human Rights, charging Westchester County Medical Center (WCMC) with employment discrimination. The division conducted a hearing and concluded that Doe was illegally denied employment as a pharmacist because of a handicap. WCMC faced the choice of either hiring Doe or being denied federal funding. The medical center stalled, claiming that Doe did not have a handicap but was rather a threat to patient safety. The progress of the case through the legal system resulted in a landmark decision that human immunodeficiency virus (HIV) infection was a handicap and that persons with HIV infection were therefore protected under existing laws preventing employment discrimination on the basis of that handicap. The civil rights impact of this decision is incalculable. How the US public health system, which is invisible to most Americans, worked to support Doe's civil rights is part of this story.

BACKGROUND

I learned about John Doe when I served as one of the expert witnesses in the case's administrative court hearing in 1991, but I never knew the details of the case until more than twenty years later. As part of the background for this book, I read the judge's decision (1) and the affirmation of the judge's decision by a three-judge panel of the Civil Rights Reviewing Authority (2). I was surprised to learn that, before my testimony, I had not received important information about the case that was available at the time. Because even now the details of the story are sketchy, I tried to contact Doe for an interview through his lawyer, Evan Wolfson, who during the hearing worked with Lambda Legal. Wolfson responded, in 2014, that he had lost contact with Doe many years ago and could not contact him on my behalf.

John Doe had pursued this case for more than six years despite the risk of his identity's being exposed and the great risk of being subjected to backlash, ridicule, and lifelong employment discrimination were the case unsuccessful. Given the climate at the time—marked by widespread fear and hatred of persons with HIV infection or AIDS—Doe showed remarkable courage. One can understand why the anonymous term John Doe was used to protect his privacy.

LEGAL ISSUES

The case was initiated before 1990 and was therefore governed by section 504 of the Rehabilitation Act of 1973. This act states that it is unlawful for a program or activity that receives federal financial assistance to discriminate against an otherwise-qualified person with a handicap solely on the basis of that handicap. The Americans with Disabilities Act, passed by the US Congress in 1990 (during the legal proceedings of this case), provides even greater protection against employment discrimination for persons with disabilities.

MEDICAL DETECTIVES AS EXPERT WITNESSES

Because CDC epidemiologists frequently become experts in particular diseases, especially new or rare ones, they are sought after to be expert witnesses in medical malpractice and other medically related lawsuits. CDC tries to protect its employees as much as possible from testimony unless it is clearly in the interest of the public's health. Depending on the circumstances, expert witnesses may be well paid, and whichever side has the most resources usually has the best witnesses. As a federal government employee, however, a CDC physician cannot accept payment for serving as an expert witness, and so there is no financial motivation to testify.

You may recall the movie *The Verdict*, in which a Catholic hospital is sued for malpractice. Paul Newman, who plays the plaintiff's lawyer, believes he has locked in one of the hospital doctors as a witness. But he soon discovers that the defendants have paid the physician off, and the only expert witness he can get is a doctor with no particular expertise in the medical issue at hand and little credibility. In real life, casting doubt on the credentials and opinions of expert witnesses is a blood sport between opposing legal counsels. Lawyers spend a great deal of time and money searching the background of opposing witnesses, scrutinizing their publications and public statements, malpractice claims, and previous testimony. They even look for any kind of witness indiscretion, such as drunken driving arrests. Any "dirt" that is dug up is fair game and can be used to embarrass, humiliate, or otherwise discredit the witness. At the time of John Doe's hearing, in 1991, no Internet existed to facilitate the search, so legal assistants or even the lawyers themselves conducted research on medical experts.

HHS v. WCMC was heard before Judge Steven T. Kessel in a New York City courtroom in August 1991. This was a hearing, not a trial, so there was no jury present. The judge reviewed the evidence provided by each side and made the final decision. An administrative law judge such as Kessel has the power to make a number of prehearing decisions. One decision made in this case was to limit the number of expert witnesses. CDC and the National Institutes of Health (NIH) are both Health and Human Services (HHS) agencies, and each agency was asked to provide only one expert witness for the hearing. I was the CDC witness, and David Henderson, MD, was the NIH witness. The defense team witness was Peter Mansell, MD, an oncologist in private practice in Houston. Dr. Henderson and I were both members of the Commissioned Corps of the Public Health Service, a uniformed service headed by the US surgeon general, and we were told to wear our uniforms. Because we both held ranks of captain (equivalent to Navy captain), HHS assumed that the uniforms would enhance our authoritative appearance.

The CDC director at the time told me that I would be the expert witness but would not say why I was chosen. I was but one of many CDC scientists with experience in examining and interpreting HIV/AIDS epidemiologic data. However, I had just stepped down as the associate director for science, a position that required top-secret security clearance and a background investigation by the Federal Bureau of Investigation (FBI). My security clearance might have been a factor in my selection as the expert witness, as the defense counsel could hardly do a more thorough background check than the FBI (although, in hindsight, this might have been wishful thinking). Incidentally, during that background check, a neighbor whom I barely knew called and told me that the FBI had contacted him for an interview about me. He was upset because he thought I had given his name to the FBI as a personal reference. I told him I had not given his name to the FBI, explained the reason for the background check, and offered my apologies. He called back a few weeks later and said that he had told the FBI during the interview that he disapproved of me because I had not changed my name when I got married. Apparently, the FBI did not have a problem with the neighbor's report because I survived the background check.

The HHS Office of General Counsel in Washington, DC, informed me that Michael Astrue, the general counsel at the time, would be the lead attorney for the case. CDC also has an Office of General Counsel, and one of its lawyers, Verla Neslund, was assigned to help me prepare for the hearing. Wanda Jones, DrPH, a CDC scientist in the HIV/AIDS program, was an HHS consultant, so it was a three-woman CDC team, very unusual at that time.

WHAT I KNEW BEFORE TESTIMONY

HHS had selected this particular case as a "test case," that is, a case with the purpose of setting a precedent. The goal was for the court to determine that HIV infection was a handicap covered by the 1973 Rehabilitation Act.

About John Doe

John Doe was a registered pharmacist licensed to practice in New York State. He was working as a pharmacist at another hospital when he applied for a position at WCMC. After an interview with WCMC personnel in October 1986, he was told that he would be hired after passing a preemployment physical examination, and that he should expect to start work in December. The position he had applied for was the midnight to 8:00 a.m. shift in the main pharmacy, which included a 5 percent higher pay differential. In December 1986, Doe went to WCMC for his preemployment physical. Somehow, the physician who performed the examination found out that Doe was HIV positive. Doe himself did not reveal his status, and he could not have been tested for HIV without his signed consent, so something very unusual must have occurred.

The blood test for HIV (antibody) was first licensed in 1985 amid a great deal of controversy concerning who should be tested and why. Because no effective treatment for HIV infection yet existed, why should people be tested? A positive test would surely be a stigma, resulting in a severe downside for the person tested, with little tangible benefit. Many gay-rights organizations opposed testing on these grounds. The greatest public health benefit from the test would have been its use in the blood supply industry to screen donors and eliminate all HIV-positive blood. But even here controversy existed. Did the screening agencies have to report to public health agencies the names of volunteer blood donors who tested HIV positive? If so, would such reporting significantly reduce the number of blood donor volunteers and thus endanger the nation's blood supply? There were many more reasons for and against HIV testing. For a person at risk, knowing his or her HIV status would hopefully lead to safe sexual behavior, preventing transmission to partners. It would also help healthcare providers give advice on the many associated health issues and potential therapies for HIV infection.

Doe must have gotten tested voluntarily sometime between 1985 and 1986, and a worst-case scenario ensued. WCMC refused to employ him, and he was "outed" as HIV positive. WCMC never contacted Doe again. There was no job offer, nor did he receive notification that he would not be hired. This outcome was exactly why so many civil rights activists at that time advised against HIV testing.

Before my testimony, I did not know how the WCMC examining physician found out Doe was HIV positive nor how Doe had in turn learned that the physician had discovered Doe's HIV status. But Doe must have, because in December 1986, he filed a complaint at the State Division of Human Rights charging that he was not hired for the pharmacist job solely because he had HIV infection (3).

About Westchester County Medical Center

WCMC's attorneys responded to Doe's complaint in February 1987, stating that they declined to hire Doe for "medical reasons which they considered to be compelling," and rejected the claim that Doe was handicapped (4). WCMC is a hospital and medical center that, between 1986 and 1991, annually treated more than 22,000 inpatients and over 100,000 outpatients. It was also a tertiary- and acute-care medical center serving a seven-county area of New York State known as the mid-Hudson Valley. It has an open-heart surgery center, organ transplant services, a comprehensive cancer care center, a pediatric intensive care unit, and a level-1 trauma center. At the time of the lawsuit, its annual budget was $252 million. Approximately 60 percent of WCMC's patients received services that were reimbursed by Medicare or Medicaid. WCMC received $107 million annually, or more than 40 percent of its budget from federal funds. If this support were terminated, it would be a crippling financial blow to the medical center. The WCMC pharmacy employed forty pharmacists, including supervisors, to work in their main and satellite pharmacies throughout the medical center campus. The main pharmacy is open 24 hours a day, 365 days a year. The duties of all pharmacists and supervisors include the preparation of parenteral products, that is, those administered to patients by injection, such as cancer drugs and nutritional supplements.

In November 1987, when it became clear that HHS was going to take action to terminate the medical center's federal funding, WCMC offered Doe a compromise, a position in a satellite pharmacy with the restriction that he could not prepare parenteral products. WCMC outlined a scenario in which the pharmacist, while preparing parental products, could prick his finger when using a syringe and needle and not realize it. If his blood were on the needle, it might then contaminate the parenteral medications that he was preparing, and therefore HIV could be *indirectly* transmitted to the patient. Because pharmacists at the hospital did not provide direct patient care, there was no risk of *direct* HIV transmission from pharmacist to patient.

Both HHS and Doe rejected the offer as a solution to the discrimination complaint. Doe would not be able to work at the main pharmacy; therefore he was ineligible for the midnight to 8:00 a.m. shift and its accompanying 5 percent pay differential. In addition,

Doe would not be eligible for a supervisory position, because supervisors were required at times to prepare parenteral products. The case dragged on in a stalemate until December 1990, when HHS filed an action to terminate federal funding to WCMC. The WCMC attorneys responded immediately, requesting an administrative law judge hearing. The request was granted, and the hearing was held from August 5 to 12, 1991, in a New York City courtroom.

PREPARATION AND TESTIMONY

Our CDC team's best guess was that the defense attorneys would focus on what evidence existed about the risk of HIV and any other infection in the healthcare setting, either from the healthcare worker to the patient or the patient to the healthcare worker. I particularly searched the medical literature for even one case of a hospital-acquired infection in which a pharmacist was found to be the cause of the infection. I found none.

Within two years of the first case reports of AIDS, all the modes of transmission of HIV infection had been established: sexual intercourse, transfusion of blood or blood products, intravenous drug use with contaminated needles, and transmission from mother to infant during delivery or breast-feeding. These modes of transmission were similar to those for hepatitis B, and because healthcare workers were at considerable occupational risk for hepatitis B infection, the concern was that they might also be at increased risk for HIV infection. So CDC began a nationwide surveillance study in 1983 of healthcare workers who had needlestick or exposures from blood or body fluids of AIDS patients to determine their risk of developing HIV infection after exposure. After three years of study, the results showed that the risk of transmission was a relatively low 0.35 percent, compared to the 19 to 27 percent risk for hepatitis B infection from exposure to a hepatitis B needlestick (5). Other studies confirmed this lower risk. In fact, Dr. Henderson, the NIH expert witness, published a study showing that no HIV infections occurred in 332 NIH Clinical Center workers who had been exposed to blood or body fluids from AIDS patients (6).

As of 2008, there was only one documented case in the United States of a healthcare worker transmitting HIV infection to patients: that of a dentist to patients during invasive dental work (7).

I was the first expert witness to testify. After my first day on the stand, the defense attorney told the judge that he predicted he would need my testimony for another two or three days. The judge refused, stating that this estimate was excessive, and said he would only allow for one more day of my testimony. The defense attorney asked if I had reviewed John Doe's medical record provided to all expert witnesses in advance by the defense. I had. He asked me what I thought of it. The record contained only two laboratory reports and no physician's notes. One report contained the results of a blood screen performed at WCMC for new employees, and the results were normal. The other was a test for CD4 lymphocytes, white blood cells that are part of the immune system and that are the particular cells attacked and destroyed by HIV. Because CD4 counts decrease as untreated HIV infection progresses, they are used to follow the status of the immune system in patients with HIV infection. Noticeably absent from the record was an HIV test. The defense attorney asked if I remembered what Doe's CD4 count was. I replied that I did not. He expressed incredulity.

"Why wouldn't you remember?" he asked. I explained that no standardized, Food and Drug Administration–licensed laboratory test for CD4 counts existed and that the laboratory report in Doe's record had no indication what laboratory performed the test or what the normal values for that laboratory were. As a result, I could not interpret the test results. The attorney discontinued this line of questioning. Most of his subsequent questions were about the published reports of the risk for HIV infection in the healthcare setting.

On my second day on the stand, the lead counsel said to me, "I give up. Why are you wearing that uniform?" My uniform must have irked him, giving credibility to the idea that the uniform had *some* positive effect for the plaintiff's side.

Before lunch on that day, the defense lawyer stated that published reports showed considerable differences in the estimated risk of HIV transmission in healthcare settings. He referred to the results in two different publications, and I asked to see them. I explained to him that the data from one study were presented in decimals and the other in percentages, but that they were essentially equivalent risks. At lunch, my team colleagues, Ms. Neslund and Dr. Jones, who had been in the courtroom, commented that my explanation about the differences in the two studies was technically correct, but they weren't sure that my answer was clear enough for the judge to understand. They suggested that, if the issue came up again, I address the judge with my answer and not the lead counsel. (We believed that the lawyers knew the studies gave the same result but were trying to create doubt in the judge's mind.) The discussions over the publications continued in the courtroom in the afternoon, and this time I addressed the judge, pointing out that the risks found were the same in both studies, only expressed differently. The judge then asked me several questions, and it was clear he understood. It was great to have my colleagues in the courtroom to help me clarify that important issue.

The last series of questions addressed to me were about how sure I was that a pharmacist with HIV infection could not indirectly infect a patient by inadvertently contaminating parenteral medications with his blood.

"Could this never happen?" the defense attorney asked. I answered with the adage I had learned in medical school, "Never say never in medicine." But I pointed out that the likelihood that a pharmacist would prick himself with a needle and not know or see the blood was extremely small, and the likelihood that HIV could live in parenteral solutions was unknown but also very small. (To survive, HIV needs living cells, which parenteral solutions do not have.) I answered that the risk of transmission was extremely small but incalculable. The lawyer asked whether, even with this small risk, the hospital shouldn't be 100 percent sure, to protect the patients, and thus deny the pharmacist the job.

Mr. Astrue, general counsel for HHS, objected to the continued "what-if" questions, and to the constructed scenarios of possible routes of transmission. The judge agreed, and my testimony was soon over. I would have loved to be present at the testimony of the other two expert witnesses, but expert witnesses are only permitted in court for their own testimony.

Judge Kessel decided the case for HHS and determined that federal funding for WCMC should be terminated. He stated that he based his decision on the testimony of HHS expert witnesses because they are "not only medical experts but are charged with public health responsibilities." The area in which the HHS witnesses and defense witness disagreed was on the public health implications of the evidence. Both Drs. Guinan and Henderson, he said, testified that the risk that Doe might infect a patient with HIV through his preparation of parenteral products was so small as to be unquantifiable. The opposing witness, Dr. Mansell, had agreed that the risk was small but that no matter how small the risk Doe should not be allowed to prepare parenteral products.

Judge Kessel stated, "I find these [HHS] experts' conclusions to be credible and to be buttressed strongly by the evidence which they relied on. The evidence establishes that there has never been a single episode documented of a pharmacist transmitting either HIV or hepatitis B through a contaminated parenteral product" (1).

Without CDC's surveillance studies, there would have been insufficient evidence to decide the case. These studies of the risk of HIV transmission in the workplace were started in 1983, two years after the first reported AIDS cases (8), when there was no CDC AIDS budget. In an example of how the public health system worked despite the deplorable lack of HIV funding, the studies were conducted by 10 CDC investigators and cooperating investigators from 335 institutions nationwide, who followed over 1,600 healthcare workers who had needlesticks that were contaminated with blood from HIV/AIDS patients (9). These studies provided information on how HIV is transmitted and how exposures occurred. These data were used to improve healthcare workers' safety by providing infection-control guidelines and eventually led to the redesign of sharp instruments. These improvements reduced blood exposure, which is the single greatest risk of infection for healthcare workers. So the surveillance data also led to improved prevention of occupationally acquired HIV infection.

After the decision was announced, the *New York Times* reported on the case. "This is an important precedent. It is the first civil rights enforcement action based on HIV discrimination by any federal agency," Astrue was quoted as saying. The decision meant that "the federal government will not tolerate discriminatory activity for the disabled in general, and specifically for individuals with HIV" (10). WCMC appealed to the HHS Civil Rights Reviewing Authority, which reviewed the case and affirmed Judge Kessel's decision in September 1992 (2).

On January 11, 1993, HHS announced in a press release that WCMC had agreed to "comply with Section 504 of the Rehabilitation Act of 1973 and all terms of a Compliance Agreement. The medical center will offer Doe an unrestricted full time position as a hospital pharmacist with retroactive seniority to Dec 1986 and will provide him with back pay and a lump sum payment for other employee benefits" (11). Additionally, the report stated, "the Medical Center will adopt a statement of non-discrimination in which it explicitly encourages persons with AIDS and HIV infection to participate as fully as possible in all of the medical center's programs and activities." How wonderful!

A spokesperson for WCMC said it was somewhat disconcerting for the hospital to "be painted by some people as having some sort of phobia about HIV. We are one of the few AIDS management centers designated by the NY State Health Department and the only one in Westchester County. We are very sensitive to the needs of AIDS patients. To intimate anything less is an injustice (10)."

EPILOGUE

I recently learned from the narrative in the judge's decision and the civil rights authority review of the decision that, before applying for the position, Doe had been under the care of a WCMC physician at the infectious diseases clinic. Doe's personal physician had tested him for HIV, and the positive results were in Doe's medical record at WCMC. When Doe arrived for his preemployment physical, a healthcare worker recognized him as a clinic patient and told the examining physician. Doe's records were illegally retrieved and the positive HIV test results found—an egregious break in confidentiality of patient medical records. The examining physician told Doe he had found Doe's medical record with the positive HIV test results and believed he had AIDS and would not recommend him for employment. Neither Doe's personal physician nor his medical record supported the AIDS diagnosis, and indeed Doe did not have a condition that fit the CDC case definition for AIDS. This discrepancy—and the fact that Doe's records had been obtained illegally—may explain why there was no HIV test result in Doe's medical record that was provided to expert witnesses. These facts also clarify why the attorney was so focused on the CD4 test results during my testimony. Very low CD4 counts are supportive of an

AIDS diagnosis. Fortunately, I had not remembered Doe's CD4 count. Who knows how the defense obtained these test results.

At the 1987 hearing on Doe's complaint, *Doe v. WCMC*, two WCMC physicians—an oncologist and a pathologist—testified that Doe constituted a risk for transmission of HIV to patients (12). But another physician, Gary Wormser, MD—who was chief of the WCMC infectious diseases clinic, the director of the AIDS unit, and a leading AIDS researcher—testified *against* WCMC at that hearing (13). Dr. Wormser believed that Doe would not be a threat to patient safety if he were hired. WCMC's decision to disregard its own expert HIV/AIDS researcher and continue the legal action is an example of the fear and superstition that overruled the clinical expertise and published findings of the time. But such discrimination about HIV and AIDS was prevalent at that time. It is comparable to fears today about Ebola virus in West Africa, where an epidemic is occurring, and also in the United States, where the first Ebola cases occurred in 2014. It is difficult to exaggerate the spread of fear and myths in these chaotic situations.

I recently contacted Dr. Wormser to discuss John Doe's case. He and I had worked together on some early AIDS cases in New York, and we also were classmates in medical school. (However, I never knew that he had testified at the original hearing.) He said he remembered how unhappy the hospital was about his testimony. Knowing that this was a considerable understatement, I congratulated him on having the courage to testify. But he survived, and still leads the WCMC infectious diseases unit. He is also a professor of medicine and pharmacology at New York Medical College.

Although Doe said in a statement that he would accept the pharmacist's position at WCMC, it is not known whether he did. Doe added that the outcome had been worth the fight (14).

Thank you, John Doe.

ELEVEN

The Milk Industry Challenges CDC
over the Source of a Listeriosis Outbreak

BACK in 1985, I had been appointed associate director for science at CDC. One of my responsibilities in that position was to coordinate responses to challenges to the scientific publications that emanated from CDC. During my first year in that position, we faced a formidable challenge from the milk industry about a listeriosis outbreak that CDC had investigated.

How could pasteurized milk be the source of a *Listeria monocytogenes* outbreak? The process of pasteurization, bringing milk to a high temperature for a short period of time, was specifically designed to kill bacterial organisms. But that is what a medical detective—CDC Epidemic Intelligence Service (EIS) officer David Fleming, MD—and his team found in a 1983 outbreak of listeriosis in Massachusetts (1).

The outbreak included forty-nine patients. All were hospitalized, and fourteen of them died. Seven of the cases were in mother/infant pairs, and forty-two occurred in immunosuppressed adults. This cohort of patients was characteristic of human *Listeria* infection, which attacks those with a compromised immune system. *Listeria* organisms also infect cows, causing encephalitis and uterine infection, which can result in an aborted pregnancy.

Infected cows can shed the bacteria in their milk, but until Dr. Fleming's study, human *Listeria* infection had not been shown to be transmitted through pasteurized milk. The results of Fleming's investigation were published in the *New England Journal of Medicine*, one of the most prestigious medical journals in the world (1). Yet the outbreak was puzzling. Although the epidemiologic investigation included two case-control studies that linked the infection to drinking a specific brand of pasteurized milk, exactly how the milk got contaminated was unclear. And although many samples were tested, the organism was never found in the suspected brand of milk, so there was no incontrovertible evidence, or "smoking gun." But by the time the milk was implicated as the source and the milk samples were tested, the epidemic was over, and the milk was unlikely to still be contaminated.

The milk lobby, which consists of a formidable coalition of giant milk companies and dairies, decided along with their congressional allies to challenge CDC on the study. They essentially created a "dream team" to work against CDC.

First, they retained Elliot Richardson as one of their lawyers. Richardson had served as the US attorney general in 1973, when President Nixon ordered him to fire the special prosecutor investigating the Watergate scandal. Richardson resigned rather than carry out the president's orders, and became one of the few who emerged from the Nixon administration as a man of integrity. He also had excellent credentials, having graduated from Harvard University and Harvard Law School, where he was editor and president of the *Harvard Law Review*. Between college and law school, Richardson served in the US Army infantry during the Normandy Invasion of World War II, receiving numerous decorations, including the Purple Heart. But this wasn't all. Richardson had also served in four different cabinet-level positions within the US government, including secretary of the Department of Health Education and Welfare (1970–73). And did I mention that he looked like Gregory Peck?

The medical team was led by a nationally known infectious diseases expert, epidemiologist and Harvard professor of medicine Ed

Kass, MD, PhD, and the equally famous Alex Langmuir, MD, who had been CDC's chief epidemiologist from 1948 to 1970. In 1951, Dr. Langmuir had convinced Congress to fund the EIS to train physicians and other scientists to identify, investigate, and control epidemics throughout the nation. Langmuir had developed the whole concept of infectious disease surveillance, epidemic investigation, and control. Imagine having Langmuir on the side of the milk industry opposing CDC. Quite a lineup!

And who was at CDC to face this dream team? By then, both Dave Fleming and Art Reingold, MD, the lead and senior authors, respectively, of the *New England Journal of Medicine* article, had left CDC. Claire Broome, MD, also a senior author and chief of the special pathogens unit that conducted the *Listeria* investigation, became the lead scientist for the defense. James Mason, MD, DrPH, director of CDC, and I rounded out the CDC team.

Through a Freedom of Information Act request, the milk industries' medical team had asked CDC to provide all original data from the case-control studies, including the original forms completed for each case and control and the calculations used for the results in the published study. They then hired a group of expert consultants to review the data and check all calculations.

In late 1986 and early 1987, the Health and Human Services (HHS) secretary summoned the CDC director to Washington, DC, to discuss the study with representatives of the milk industry. Claire Broome and Walter Dowdle, PhD, deputy director of CDC, attended the meeting at the office of Assistant Secretary of Health Robert Windom, MD.

Eliot Richardson and his entourage presented to Dr. Windom and the two CDC scientists the results of their team's review of the study that linked pasteurized milk to the listeriosis outbreak. Richardson stated that errors were found in the coding of data that would invalidate the study and concluded that the "data were obviously cooked." Richardson then asked Windom to have CDC recall the paper from the *New England Journal of Medicine* and implied that the coding errors were deliberate. (If true, it would imply that the scientists were guilty of misconduct in science, a very serious charge.) This was a proverbial bombshell for CDC. Because the details of the errors were not provided, Dowdle and Broome could do little but sit silently through the accusations. On their return to Atlanta, I was briefed on the situation.

Dr. Broome requested the details of the medical team's review. She and her staff agreed that two coding errors had occurred: two of the controls in the case-control studies had not answered the question of whether they had drunk milk. Instead of being coded as "not answered," they had instead been coded as "no." Broome recalculated the data using the correct coding and found that the results did not change; the odds ratios remained the same. Despite the coding error, drinking pasteurized milk from this particular brand of milk was still statistically significantly related to developing *Listeria* infection.

Broome felt vindicated. Not only were the study results sound, but also the charge of misconduct in science was refuted, as it was extremely unlikely that any scientist would deliberately miscode data that would produce the same results had they been coded correctly.

Even so, the political pressure was on from the lawyers. Calls from HHS to the CDC director continued with the question "When will the article be retracted from the medical journal?" This dispute would not be settled easily with sound science.

I suggested to the CDC director that we convene a panel of epidemiologists and biostatisticians from different parts of CDC to review the published study, the charges, and Dr. Broome's response, and then make a recommendation for a course of action. A panel of five senior epidemiologists was selected. All the information was given to the panelists, and a meeting was to be convened within two weeks.

In the meantime, I received a call from Dr. Alex Langmuir, who was referred to me from the director's office. He had wanted a private meeting with the CDC director. (Dr. Mason had been an EIS officer under Langmuir's direction.) He was told that I was handling the issue for CDC and to call me. He was not pleased that he had been refused a meeting with Dr. Mason, and he wasn't sure that I was high enough in the CDC hierarchy for him to spend his time with. I had never met him, although I certainly knew who he was. Langmuir was a veritable legend at CDC.

He told me that he had talked to a number of his friends at CDC, and they all had told him the same thing: he had to work with me. He asked if we could set up a meeting. I invited him to the panel meeting and also invited Dr. Kass and the expert consultants who had reviewed the study. CDC did not know the composition of their review team, and after a long discussion, Langmuir neither revealed any names nor made any promises to bring them to the meeting.

Langmuir arrived alone to the meeting, seemingly brimming with confidence. Besides the panel members, the other attendees included Broome and me and a representative from CDC's General Counsel's office. Langmuir knew many of the attendees and was quite cordial. After a thorough discussion by panel members, Dr. Langmuir stated his position that the coding errors were deliberate and the study should be retracted from the journal. When asked why the authors would falsify the coding if it did not change the results, he responded that the authors wanted to have the study published in a prestigious journal.

A discussion with a good deal of emotional intensity ensued. One panel member asked rather heatedly, "Alex, did you hear that the error did not change the results?" Langmuir disregarded the question and held his ground. I asked each panel member to make a statement of his conclusion and to recommend whether or not the study should be retracted. The panel members were unanimous in declaring the study sound and recommending against retraction.

I wrote a summary of the meeting and sent it to Jim Mason, who forwarded it to HHS. I assumed that this would be the end of the story, but it was not. There was a great deal of pressure on Mason for a private meeting with Drs. Kass and Langmuir. Eventually, Dr. Mason agreed to meet with them, but only if I were included. I asked that Verla Neslund from CDC's General Counsel also attend because she had been advising me on the legal aspects of defending CDC.

The meeting took place in the director's office. Dr. Kass took the lead. He stated that his primary concern was how harmful it would be to CDC's reputation if it were sued for misconduct in science. Dr. Mason replied that his associate director for science had advised him that the study was sound and he would not recommend retraction. Kass then asked me a series of questions that had little to do with the study. He said he was not taking any money for his part in the lawsuit and he was putting his reputation on the line because of the seriousness of the CDC error. He asked me to think of how CDC's reputation would be damaged forever.

Verla Neslund then spoke up. She said, "Don't worry about CDC's reputation; that's our job. We are not worried about being sued. We've been sued before and know how to deal with it." There was silence. The meeting was over. Afterward, I said goodbye to Dr. Langmuir, who replied, "See you in court."

I told Claire Broome that she had to send a letter to the *New England Journal of Medicine* with notification of the correction of the coding error. She thought it unnecessary, but I insisted. She wrote the letter and received a response from the editor, who expressed confusion about why a formal correction was needed when it did not change the results. In the end, no correction was printed. I was thinking ahead to the trial and was just grateful to get the editor's reply, which supported our case.

As months went by, the lawsuits against the grocery chain filed by the affected patients in the outbreak were bound for trial. During this time we also learned that Dr. Kass had a terminal illness. Before he died in 1990, he spent time giving depositions for the case to the milk lobby lawyers. Dr. Fleming, who led the epidemic investigation, was among the last to be deposed. Within a short time after his testimony, the lawyers announced that the lawsuits from the patients would be settled. Whether it was his testimony or other factors that pushed the lawyers to make this decision is unknown. The milk industry did not move forward with the lawsuit against CDC. We were all relieved that we did not have to testify. And the medical detective Dave Fleming eventually became the deputy director of CDC.

In 2007, another listeriosis outbreak linked to pasteurized milk occurred in Massachusetts, but this time the epidemic strain of *Listeria* was found in the milk. Evidence suggested that the milk had been contaminated in the dairy after pasteurization (2).

TWELVE

On Getting AIDS from a Toilet Seat
and Other STD Myths and Taboos

MYTHS of how one acquires a sexually transmitted disease (STD) have persisted for centuries. And now, many years after I left CDC and forged another career in Nevada as the state's health officer and then founding dean of the School of Public Health at the University of Nevada, Las Vegas, I am amazed and somewhat disheartened that these myths persist as strongly as ever.

A look at a 2009 national survey on knowledge about human immunodeficiency virus (HIV) transmission illustrates the point: 17 percent of respondents believed transmission can occur from contact with a toilet seat (1). This belief persists despite the evidence: highly trained public health epidemiologists in every state in the United States have tracked the source of infection of more than a million HIV/AIDS patients for thirty-four years, and as of 2015 not a single case has been traced to a toilet seat. Yet myth often trumps scientific evidence.

In 1957, when the Venereal Diseases Division was transferred from the Public Health Service in Washington, DC, to CDC in Atlanta, it brought with it a cadre of workers called public health advisors (PHAs), who were specially trained in tracking the source and spread of STDs (2). PHAs worked within state health departments to assist in the control of STDs and to help set up surveillance systems for syphilis and gonorrhea. Between 1958 and 1981 (when AIDS emerged), PHAs tracked the source of infection of millions of cases of syphilis and gonorrhea and, again, not one was traced to a toilet seat.

When I was growing up in New York City in the fifties, each subway car had city health department ads warning of the dangers of syphilis and gonorrhea. One day, I asked an older friend what the ads meant. She whispered that they were about diseases that one "caught" from subway bathrooms and warned me never to even say those "awful words." A taboo still exists about them. Sometimes I think it would be more acceptable at a social gathering for me to use the "F word" than to talk about syphilis or gonorrhea.

When I joined CDC's STD unit in 1978, I learned a great deal from PHAs about their fascinating experiences in tracking the source of STDs. In the early years of the AIDS epidemic, I learned just how harmful the toilet myth and other associated jokes could be.

One day, a reporter from CNN called to ask my opinion on an ongoing controversy. Female workers at a small unit of an insurance company in Chicago were picketing the company because they were forced to use a bathroom with only one toilet. The women believed that one of their co-workers had AIDS, and they did not want to use the same toilet for fear of contracting the disease. The physician medical director of the company supported the women in their protest. I was stunned. I responded that no case of AIDS had ever been traced to a toilet seat and expressed my concern about CNN's airing the story. The woman whose co-workers thought had AIDS was not only being unfairly targeted but also being publicly humiliated—whether she had AIDS or not.

The next day the reporter called back. The story had been carried in a Chicago newspaper, and CNN wanted me to give my opinion on camera. I declined because I believed it would be just another sideshow in the regrettably bad early media coverage of AIDS. But CNN persisted in its request, and the CDC media unit persuaded me to do the interview, although I was not happy about

it. During the interview, the reporter asked whether I was absolutely sure one could not get AIDS from a toilet seat. I answered
with a line that a PHA had given me: "The only way I know of that
you can get AIDS from a toilet seat is if you sit down on it before
someone else gets up." With that, the interview was over. My response was somewhat flippant, and I regretted saying it (at least on
television). I never saw the news clip, but many people did. I have
often seen my quote in slide or PowerPoint presentations at medical meetings. A colleague once told me that this line would be my
epitaph.

MYTHS THAT PERSIST

Before the germ theory of disease was recognized in the early nineteenth century, STDs were believed to be caused by either "bad
humors" in the air or by God as a punishment for sin. By the early
twentieth century, both the cause of syphilis (*Treponema pallidum*,
a bacterial spirochete) and its primary transmission through sexual
intercourse were well established. But the belief that syphilis and
other STDs were a punishment from God persisted. STDs were
perceived to be moral failures rather than health issues, and little
sympathy existed for those afflicted. The shame and vilification of
those with syphilis led many patients to hide their infection. Even
if they sought help, many physicians refused to treat them.

Another common belief in the United States throughout the
early twentieth century was that fear of contracting syphilis was a
strong deterrent to "immoral" sexual behavior. Many physicians
held this belief, even one of the founding four professors at the
great Johns Hopkins Hospital, which had one of the first specialty
clinics for syphilis treatment. Dr. Howard A. Kelly, professor of
gynecology and obstetrics, wrote, "I believe that if we could in an
instant eradicate the diseases [STDs] we would also forget at once
the moral side of the question, and would then, in one short gener-

ation, fall wholly under the domination of the animal passions, becoming grossly and universally immoral" (3). Following this line of reasoning, physicians who treated syphilis were promoting "sin with impunity," thereby contributing to the perceived increase in moral depravity of the population. The secrecy, stigma, shame, and lack of treatment for syphilis laid the groundwork for the worst syphilis epidemic in US history, in the late 1920s through the 1930s. The epidemic was ample evidence that fear of contracting syphilis did not result in a high rate of celibacy. But the United States has continued to promote this belief into the twenty-first century, as is evident through government-sponsored "abstinence only" sex education programs based on the idea that fear of STDs and unplanned pregnancy will scare teens into celibacy. None of these programs has shown evidence of effectiveness.

In his book *No Magic Bullet*, Allan M. Brandt described the social history of venereal disease in the United States from 1880 to 1985 (4). The magic bullet was a concept, advanced by Dr. Paul Ehrlich, Nobel laureate in medicine in 1908, that if a substance could be found that killed the disease-causing organism but was safe for the patient, then treatment of the afflicted patients would eventually eliminate the disease from the population. Ehrlich and coworkers began a search for a magic bullet to kill the syphilis spirochete. After testing 605 possibilities, they found "compound 606," or arsphenamine (eventually named Salvarsan), which was effective for curing syphilis in rabbits. By 1910, Salvarsan was found to cure syphilis in patients and was soon mass-produced in Germany, becoming the most widely prescribed drug in the world. Great Britain and Scandinavian countries began government-funded national programs with free clinics for syphilis diagnoses and Salvarsan treatment. These health initiatives, unburdened by moral overtones, resulted in a dramatic decrease in syphilis in these countries. By contrast, the disease rates soared in the United States (5).

Brandt maintained that continuing controversies throughout the twentieth century—about religious beliefs, sexual mores, whether STDs were medical or moral issues, and whether STD control was a personal or societal responsibility—severely hampered syphilis control efforts. He concluded that if we continue the same approach—that is, implying that certain sexual behaviors are sinful, and STDs are the punishment—it will take much more than magic bullets to eliminate STDs (6).

The public reaction to the emerging AIDS epidemic in the 1980s eerily mirrored the response to syphilis control efforts earlier in the century. Many critics responded with statements such as "Why should public resources be spent on sinners, so they can continue their immoral lifestyle?" "Homosexuality is a sin, and AIDS is a punishment from God." "Curing AIDS would only encourage homosexuality, resulting in a breakdown of social mores."

But then the country was faced with the "innocents," people who contracted AIDS nonsexually, including those with hemophilia, recipients of contaminated blood transfusions, newborns infected by their mothers, and heterosexual partners of intravenous drug users. Should they be treated differently from those who were considered sinners? Gay activists became a major force in demanding that AIDS be recognized as a deadly national health problem rather than a moral issue.

LESSONS LEARNED FROM PROGRAMS TO ELIMINATE SYPHILIS

Many dedicated physicians, public health programs, and progressive movements in the United States worked diligently to eliminate syphilis. One of the first and most prominent was Dr. Thomas Parran, a public health physician frustrated at the lack of an organized approach to the appalling syphilis epidemic in the early twentieth century. Parran was essentially ignored until 1930, when Governor

Franklin Roosevelt appointed him as the New York State health commissioner. Parran spent much of his time trying to gather information on the burden of STDs and their associated healthcare costs. He considered syphilis the most serious public health problem for not only New York but also the entire nation.

In 1934, Parran was scheduled to give an address on CBS radio on the "state of the health of New York." A few minutes before the program began, CBS executives told Parran that he could not use the words *syphilis* or *gonorrhea* in his talk. He refused to go on the air and, angry at being censored, he released his speech to the press. Despite taboos on the use of "those words," many prominent newspapers printed the speech, causing a public furor. Parran later lamented that "among American handicaps to syphilis control is the widespread belief that nice people don't talk about syphilis, nice people don't have syphilis, and nice people shouldn't do anything about those who do have syphilis" (7). Dr. Prince Morrow, an American dermatologist, sociologist, and leader in the earlier progressive movement to control STDs in the late nineteenth and early twentieth centuries, expressed similar frustrations: "Social sentiment holds that it is a greater violation of the properties of life publicly to mention venereal disease than privately to contract it" (8).

Parran criticized the members of the New York Senate who voted against changing the name of the Department of Health's Division of Social Hygiene to the Division of Syphilis Control and especially the two senators from New York City who spoke against this change, one of them saying, "this bill would only be giving our children a new word to talk about. It is not decent or necessary." In reply, Parran "respectfully called to the attention of the senators" that 67,010 cases of syphilis (clinically and laboratory diagnosed) were reported in New York City alone in 1936. He then compared syphilis cases in that city with those in the country of Sweden, which had approximately the same population (over six million people). In 1935, New York City had over 35,000 clinical cases of syphilis; Sweden had 399. Parran wrote, "If an enemy with troops and battleships were attacking both Sweden and the U.S. and killing ninety of our citizens for every Swedish fatality, perhaps even [the senator] would be willing to mention the name of this enemy in order to rouse united public action against it" (9).

THE SYPHILIS EPIDEMIC OF THE 1930s

Franklin Roosevelt became president in 1933. Unlike many of today's political leaders, Roosevelt was interested in attacking the venereal disease problem. (Ronald Reagan, who was president when the AIDS epidemic emerged, refused to say the word *AIDS* or provide federal funding for the control of that disease until several years into his administration, when his friend Rock Hudson died from the disease.) Roosevelt appointed Parran as US surgeon general in 1936 (he served until 1948), and *Time* magazine put his picture on the October 26, 1936, cover for his efforts to control syphilis.

Parran's landmark book *Shadow on the Land: Syphilis* was published the following year. In it, he estimated that the prevalence or total number of existing syphilis cases in the United States was more than six million, and that one in ten adults either had syphilis or would get it unless the disease was brought under control. The estimated number of new cases each year (annual incidence) was 518,000.

Untreated syphilis infection lasts a lifetime and has four stages. The first stage is a painless ulcer or *chancre,* which occurs where the organism entered the skin. This chancre is full of spirochetes and can penetrate skin or mucous membranes that touch it. After a few weeks, the chancre heals spontaneously, but by then the spirochete has spread to virtually all organs of the body. Persons with syphilis may feel that they are cured, but within a few weeks, the second stage arrives, with a skin rash and aches and pains resulting from the ongoing damage to the heart and eyes, brain, liver, and kidneys. The patient's symptoms might include fever, headache, joint pain, and a rash. The rash occurs on the skin, in the mucous membranes of the mouth and genital area, and even on the palms of the hands and the soles of the feet. Wherever the rash is, its pustules are filled with tiny spirochetes, which can jump to another person's skin if touched. Then follows stage three, a period of latency, when the disease again becomes invisible but the spirochetes are internally destroying eyes, aortas, brains, and the unborn. The fourth stage (tertiary syphilis, so named because it is the third symptomatic stage) doesn't occur in all cases, but when it does, some ten to twenty years later, the symptoms include insanity, blindness, heart disease, and many other problems.

Parran estimated that, in 1937, syphilis was responsible for 15 percent of all blindness in the United States and 50 percent of children born blind, 18 percent of all deaths from heart disease, 10 percent of all insanity cases, and 60,000 babies born each year with congenital syphilis. The healthcare costs for the effects of syphilis had brought many of the states to a severe financial crisis, further straining a national economy still in the depths of the Great Depression. Parran's book was a plea to view syphilis as a public health issue that caused devastating illness rather than as a moral problem. He emphasized the effect on the family and the often-innocent wife whose husband gave her syphilis, of which she was unaware, and who then unknowingly passed it on to her newborn. Parran noted that a wet nurse with a syphilis rash could also pass syphilis on to a suckling infant. It could even be transmitted by a kiss if the chancre or rash were in the mouth. (These last examples of contracting syphilis occurred without "sinning.") Making the case that the cost of treating and eliminating syphilis would be far less than the existing healthcare costs for all stages of the disease (which were the responsibility of the state), Parran made a compelling case to view syphilis as an economic, not moral, issue. He also presented a plan to fund a syphilis elimination program.

Parran served on a committee that helped draft the Social Security Act (SSA) of 1935. The SSA contained a provision (Title VI) for an annual allocation of funds to the Public Health Service for the purpose of assisting states in establishing and maintaining adequate public health services. Parran was determined to use some of this fund for a syphilis elimination program. This would be the first time (except during wartime) that the federal government considered health as *its* responsibility. Authority for health matters is not mentioned in the US Constitution and therefore is assigned to the states (in the Tenth Amendment). The SSA did not take authority away from the states but permitted the federal government to provide states with public health funding. As a result, clinics for the diagnosis and treatment of syphilis using Salvarsan were established throughout the country. It was a slow process, as eighteen weekly injections of Salvarsan were deemed necessary for cure, and there were many toxic side effects.

But, fortuitously, in 1944, penicillin began to be mass-produced. This antibiotic was found to be so highly effective for curing all stages of syphilis with minimal side effects that it became the treatment of choice. The penicillin cure rate for syphilis was well over 90 percent, and many patients were cured with just one treatment. It is difficult to exaggerate the dramatic effect of penicillin on the syphilis epidemic. Between 1944 and 1954, the total number of syphilis case rates fell by 75 percent, and new syphilis cases were reduced by more than 90 percent. In 1957, the number of new syphilis cases fell to approximately 6,000, the lowest number recorded since surveillance began in 1941 (10).

Compared to the estimated 500,000 new syphilis cases in 1937, it seemed that Parran's dream might come true. He had estimated that it would take ten years to eliminate syphilis from the country, and the goal was clearly in sight. But as CDC later learned from the Smallpox Eradication Program, the last cases are the most elusive to find and contain. Because the syphilis program was so successful, it was assumed that it needed fewer resources. So from 1945 to 1955, funds to the Public Health Service for its venereal disease program decreased from $12 to $3 million. Syphilis cases again started climbing, and by 1961, they numbered over 18,000. Dr. William Brown, director of Venereal Disease Control at CDC, fought for more funding for all STDs, but polio was now one of the chief concerns of the public health community (and polio was not linked to sinful behavior), and there was public apathy about syphilis. The director ruefully told a reporter about Brown's Law: "As the point of eradication is approached, it is more often the program that is eradicated than the disease" (11).

In 1965, an educational consultant at CDC wrote two books on STDs, one for medical professionals and one for the public, in which he tried to educate the public to separate STDs from sin (12). But one of his books incited controversy by claiming that Christopher Columbus's end-of-life insanity was caused by syphilis. The national Columbus Day Committee was outraged that the man who "discovered" America was being slandered, and demanded that the claim be removed from future editions of the book. But this was not enough for the Knights of Columbus, who appealed to President Lyndon Johnson's special assistant, Jack Valenti. CDC was eventually required to remove any mention of Christopher Columbus from the 52,000 existing copies of the book (13). The implication was that Columbus could not have been a sinner and therefore could not have had syphilis. Despite his best intentions, the author had reemphasized, rather than diminished, the link between immoral behavior and syphilis.

Efforts to eliminate syphilis have continued, including the most recent campaigns by the surgeon general in 1999 and 2006 (14). In 2000, new syphilis cases reached their lowest level in history (about 2,000 cases), but unfortunately new cases have surged since that time, to more than 16,000 in 2013. The reasons for this resurgence of syphilis cases are complex, but they are not caused by penicillin resistance. Penicillin is still the treatment of choice for syphilis and has maintained its effectiveness for over sixty years. The most recently recognized barrier to syphilis elimination in the United States is its overlap with the AIDS epidemic (10). Each disease may enhance the transmission of the other.

There is one last disgrace regarding syphilis in the United States and Dr. Parran. Two shockingly unethical STD studies were conducted while Dr. Parran was surgeon general (15). In one—the Tuskegee study of black men with syphilis, started in 1932—the men were not treated with penicillin when it became available in the 1940s. They were only treated in 1972, when a whistleblower revealed the truth to the public. In the second study, conducted from 1946 to 1948 in Guatemala, American researchers deliberately exposed more than a thousand Guatemalans to syphilis, gonorrhea, and chancroid. This study was kept secret until 2010.

In 1997, President Bill Clinton apologized to the participants in the Tuskegee study and their families. In 2010, then–US Secretary of State Hillary Clinton and Health and Human Services Secretary Kathleen Sibelius issued a formal apology to Guatemalans.

The harm done to the participants of these studies and their families is immeasurable. Although Dr. Parran was a visionary and a pioneer for the control of STDs, these controversial studies will rightly overshadow his work and public health image forever. They will also taint public health's image—and thus public health's impact. The Tuskegee studies, for example, undoubtedly led to many black Americans' deep distrust of the public health system's messages about AIDS—a distrust that lingers to this day.

Another taboo concerns the prevention of STDs and the use of condoms. Regardless of the amount of explicit sexuality on the Internet, on television, and in movies, it is still rare to see television advertisements for condoms or for the content of television programs to mention condom use as a means of preventing STDs. Surgeon General C. Everett Koop broke the taboo on government officials using the "c-word" when he released his AIDS Report to the press, in October 1986, in which he discussed the use of condoms for preventing AIDS. An abbreviated version of this release was eventually distributed to every American household in 1988.

I gave a talk on AIDS to a medical audience sometime later and encouraged the audience to advise sexually active men and women (heterosexual and homosexual) to always carry condoms and make sure that they knew how to use them to prevent infection. A few days later, I received a call from an "investigator" for syndicated columnist Jack Anderson, a Pulitzer Prize–winning author and radio show host who was dedicated to exposing government fraud and waste. The investigator told me that Anderson was going to write a column about how CDC was wasting the government's money teaching homosexuals how to have sex with condoms, and he understood that I had given a talk on this subject recently. No amount of discussion dissuaded him, so I referred him to the director of the HIV/AIDS Program at CDC. Anderson eventually called for an investigation on how CDC spent AIDS prevention funds.

In response to the surgeon general's report, *Time* magazine dedicated a whole issue to sex education of children, and I was interviewed for it. I called the representatives of condom companies to let them know about the sex-education issue and suggested that it might be a good issue in which to place a condom ad. With two CDC colleagues, I had traveled to Alabama to tour the largest condom manufacturing plant in the country. We were impressed with the manufacturing process and the quality-control standards for the products. I thought that the time was right for the marketing of condoms. (I was relieved to learn that all condom manufacturers at the time were privately held companies. As an advocate of condom use, I was often asked if I had stock in condom companies—which would have been a conflict of interest.) On November 24, 1986, *Time*'s STD issue was published without a single condom ad. The magazine refused to accept them. The same issue *did* have a back-cover, full-page advertisement for cigarettes, a substance that has been proven to kill, but it had no room for an advertisement for a product that might save lives.

I rest my case.

REFERENCES

CHAPTER TWO

1. Foege WF. House on fire: The fight to eradicate smallpox. Berkeley: University of California Press; 2011.

CHAPTER FOUR

1. Sabin AB. Misery of recurrent herpes: What to do? New England Journal of Medicine. 1975;293:986–88.
2. Guinan ME, MacCalman J, Kern ER, et al. Topical ether in herpes simplex labialis. JAMA. 1980;243(10):1059–61.
3. Guinan ME. Session 27: Herpes simplex and EB viruses. Interscience Conference on Antimicrobial Agents and Chemotherapy. Oct. 1–4, 1978. Atlanta, GA.
4. CDC. *Pneumocystis carinii* pneumonia, San Francisco. MMWR. 1981;30: 250–52.
5. Mather AD. Mystery of AIDS begins to unravel. Infection Reporter. 1984; 1(6):1–2.
6. Mather AD. Media medicine or what's a nice doc like you doing on TV? Infection Reporter. 1989;6(9):65–67.

CHAPTER FIVE

1. How the CIA's fake vaccination campaign endangers us all. Scientific American. 2013;308(5).
2. Letter to Obama: www.virology.ws/2013/08/deans-write-to-Obama -about-CIA-vaccine-scheme-in-Pakistan.

CHAPTER SIX

1. CDC. *Pneumocystis pneumonia*—Los Angeles. MMWR. 1981;30:250–52.
2. Shilts R. And the band played on: Politics, people, and the AIDS epidemic. New York: St. Martin's Griffin; 1987.

3. Jaffe HW, Choi K, Thomas PA, et al. National case-control study of Kaposi's sarcoma and *Pneumocystis carinii* pneumonia in homosexual men: Part 1, epidemiologic results. Annals of Internal Medicine. 1983;99:145–51.

CHAPTER SEVEN

1. Guinan ME, Hardy A. Epidemiology of AIDS in women in the United States, 1981–86. JAMA. 1987; 257:2039–42.
2. Gould RD. Reassuring news about AIDS: A doctor tells why you may not be at risk. Cosmopolitan Magazine. 1988 Jan.
3. Coady E. 300 protest definition of AIDS. ACT UP group claims CDC is killing women. Atlanta Journal Constitution. 1990 Dec. 4. p. D3.

CHAPTER NINE

1. Ryan H. How to whitewash a plague. New York Times. 2013 Aug. 3.

CHAPTER TEN

1. *Department of Health and Human Services (HHS) v. Westchester County Medical Center*. DAB CR191. 1992 Apr. 20.
2. Civil Rights reviewing authority's decision on review of administrative law judge decision Westchester County Medical Center. DAB 1357. 1992 Sept. 25.
3. DAB CR191, Findings of fact and conclusions of law, finding 128.
4. Ibid., finding 129.
5. McCray E, and the Cooperative Needlestick Surveillance Group. Occupational risk of the acquired immunodeficiency syndrome among health care workers. New England Journal of Medicine. 1986;314:1127–32.
6. Henderson DK, Saah AJ, Zak BJ, et al. Risk of nosocomial infection with human T-cell lymphotropic virus type III/lymphadenopathy-associated virus in a large cohort of intensively exposed health care workers. Annals of Internal Medicine. 1986;104:644–47.
7. Henderson DK. Human immunodeficiency virus in health care settings. In: Mandell GL, Bennett JE, Dolin R. Principles and practices of infectious diseases. 7th ed. Philadelphia: Churchill, Livingstone, Elsevier; 2010. p. 3755.
8. CDC. *Pneumocystis pneumonia*—Los Angeles. MMWR. 1981;30:250–52.
9. Marcus R, and the Cooperative Needlestick Surveillance Group. Surveillance of health care workers exposed to blood from patients

infected with the human immunodeficiency virus. New England Journal of Medicine. 1988;319:1118–23.

10. Hevesi D. Hospital told to hire man with HIV. New York Times. 1992 Apr. 23.

11. HHS website. Press release January 11, 1993 [cited Aug. 27, 2014]. Available from: http://archive.hhs.gov.

12. DAB CR191, analysis FN 16.

13. Ibid., FN 17.

14. Henneberger M. Pharmacist with HIV awarded job. New York Times. 1993 Jan. 12.

CHAPTER ELEVEN

1. Fleming DW, Cochi SL, MacDonald KL, Brondum J, Hayes PS, Plikaytis BD, Audurier A, Broome CV, Reingold AL. Pasteurized milk as a vehicle of infection in an outbreak of listeriosis. New England Journal of Medicine. 1985;312(7):404–7.

2. CDC. Outbreak of *Listeria monocytogenes* infections associated with pasteurized milk from a local dairy. MMWR. 2008;57(40):1097–1100.

CHAPTER TWELVE

1. HIV stigma and discrimination in the U.S.: An evidence-based report, Nov. 2010, HIV Reports [cited Jan. 2015]. Available from: www.lambda legal.org.

2. Etheridge E. Sentinel for health: A history of the Centers for Disease Control. Berkeley and Los Angeles: University of California Press; 1992. p. 89.

3. Kelly HA, as cited in: Brandt AM. No magic bullet. New York: Oxford University Press; 1985. p. 46.

4. Brandt, No magic bullet.

5. Parran T. Shadow on the land: Syphilis. Baltimore: Waverly Press; 1937. Chapters 3, 5, 6. [Special education edition published by the American Social Hygiene Association, New York, in cooperation with Reynal & Hitchcock.]

6. Brandt, No magic bullet, p. 186.

7. Parran, Shadow on the land, p. 225.

8. Morrow PA. Publicity as a factor in venereal prophylaxis. JAMA. 1906;47(10):1246.

9. Parran, Shadow on the land, p. 226.

10. Douglas JM. Penicillin treatment of syphilis. JAMA. 2009;301(7):769–71.

11. Etheridge, Sentinel for health, p. 121.
12. Schwartz WM. Student's manual on venereal diseases: Facts about syphilis and gonorrhea. Washington, DC: American Association for Health, Physical Education, and Recreation; 1965.
13. Etheridge, Sentinel for health, p. 121–22.
14. CDC. The national plan to eliminate syphilis from the United States. Atlanta: US Department of Health and Human Services; 2006.
15. Altman L. Of medical giants, accolades and feet of clay. New York Times. 2013 Apr. 1.

INDEX